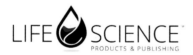

Young Living is about health without compromise. Young Living's pure, potent, natural products provide immediate, effective results without harmful side effects.

That's a real solution. That's why wellness seekers worldwide are making Young Living Essential Oils their first choice for natural healing.

THERAPEUTIC GRADE OILS

Anyone can make an essential oil that smells good, but only the world leader can deliver proven health results. Young Living's extensive experience farming, distilling, and sourcing essential oils guarantees each Young Living oil contains the optimal level of beneficial plant properties. Oils that work — that's at the core of what it means to be Young Living Therapeutic Grade™ (YLTG).

INTRODUCTION TO ESSENTIAL OILS

Essential oils, known as nature's living energy, are the natural, aromatic volatile liquids found in shrubs, flowers, trees, roots, bushes, and seeds. The distinctive components in essential oils defend plants against insects, environmental conditions, and disease. They are also vital for a plant to grow, live, evolve, and adapt to its surroundings. Essential oils are extracted from aromatic plant sources via steam distillation, and are highly concentrated and far more potent than dry herbs.

While essential oils often have a pleasant aroma, their chemical makeup is complex and their benefits vast—which makes them much more than something that simply smells good.

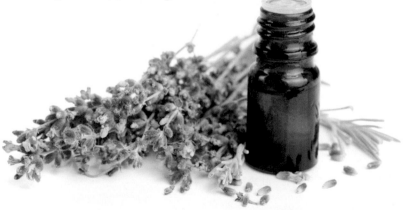

HISTORICAL USE OF ESSENTIAL OILS

Historically, essential oils have played a prominent role in everyday life. With more than 200 references to aromatics, incense, and ointments throughout the Bible, essential oils are said to be used for anointing and healing the sick. Today, essential oils are used for aromatherapy, massage therapy, emotional health, personal care, nutritional supplements, household solutions, and much more.

Young Living Essential Oils, the leading provider of essential oils, offers more than 300 essential oil singles and blends. All Young Living essential oils meet the YLTG standard. This means that every essential oil Young Living distills or sources has the optimal naturally-occurring blend of constituents to maximize the desired effect. Only YLTG essential oils should be used for the primary methods of application, which include inhalation and application.

Essential oils are considered mankind's first medicine and have been used around the world for centuries. Essential oils and other aromatics have been used in religious rituals, help support the body's natural systems, and for other physical and spiritual needs.

Research dates the use of essential oils back to 4500 B.C. Ancient Egyptians were the first to discover the potential of fragrance, and records demonstrate that oils and aromatics were used for treating illness as well as performing rituals and religious ceremonies in temples and pyramids.

According to ancient Egyptian hieroglyphics and Chinese manuscripts, priests and physicians used oils thousand of years before the time of Christ. There are more than 188 references to oils in the Bible, and some precious oils like Frankincense, Myrrh, Rosemary, Cassia, and Cinnamon were used for the anointing and healing of the sick.

DISTILLATION OF ESSENTIAL OILS

The reintroduction of essential oils into modern medicine first began during the late 19th and early 20th centuries. Since that time essential oils have been used traditionally to kill harmful germs, spiritually to balance mood, and dispel negative emotions.

The key to producing a quality essential oil is to preserve the delicate compounds of the aromatic plant through expert distillation. The proper process of steam distillation—passing steam through the plant material and condensing the steam to separate the oil from the plant—is strictly adhered to with all YLTG essential oils.

Proper temperature must be maintained throughout the distillation process. Pressure, length of time, equipment, and batch size are strictly monitored. This ensures that the naturally-occurring compounds contained in each essential oil product are of the highest and most consistent bioactive levels.

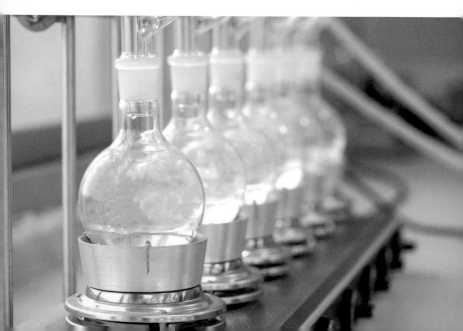

APPLICATION METHODS

(Please read the information carefully as all directions will defer to the methods outlined here.)

TOPICAL

These oils are either placed directly onto the desired location or placed on a cotton ball/cloth or on the hands and then spread over the desired area. Roll-on bottles are also available and are often used as a convenient way to apply the oil directly on the skin surface.

- **Neat:** Apply undiluted as directed to affected area.
- **Dilute 50/50:** Add 1 part essential oil(s) to 1 part V-6™ Vegetable Oil Complex.
- **Dilute 20/80:** Add 1 part essential oil(s) to 4 parts V-6™ Vegetable Oil Complex.
- **Vita Flex:** Apply 1-3 drops neat or undiluted directly on the Vita Flex points on the feet as directed.
- **Compress-Warm:** Dilute 1 part essential oil(s) with 4 parts V-6™ Vegetable Oil Complex and apply 8-10 drops on affected area. Cover with a warm, moist hand towel. Then cover the moist towel with a dry towel for 10-15 minutes.
- **Compress-Cold:** A cool, moist hand towel may also be used to create a cold compress in the same manner.
- **Body Massage:** Essential oils are typically combined with a carrier oil when used in massage. The diluted oil is spread over the desired location and then are massaged in with the hands. The oils enhance the power of the massage with their own unique properties.
- **Baths:** Essential oils are often added to baths directly or combined with bath salts to more easily dissolve in the bath water. The oils are drawn into the skin from the surrounding bath water.

ORAL

- **Gargle:** Add essential oil to purified water; shake or mix vigorously. Gargle for 30 seconds.
- **Tongue:** Let 1 drop of the essential oil or blend fall from the bottle onto the tongue, or apply with fingertip for 1 minute, then swallow.

INHALATION

- **Diffuse:** Add several drops in a cold air diffuser or in a diffuser designed for water that functions as a humidifier. Cold air diffusers are not designed to handle vegetable oils because they are thicker and may close the diffuser mechanism.
- **Inhale Directly:** Put 2-3 drops of an essential oil in the palm of one hand, rub palms together, cup hands over nose and mouth and breathe slowly. Be careful not to touch the skin near your eyes or get any oils in your eyes. If this should happen, rinse with V-6™ Vegetable Oil Complex. Do NOT rinse with water, as that will cause even more burning.

The oils listed within these pages are not a complete list of every oil you can use. For a complete list of oils and their possible uses, please reference the *Essential Oils Desk Reference.*

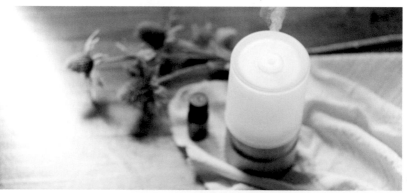

PROMOTE A HEALTHY EMOTIONAL STATE

Each essential oil boasts a complex, pleasant, and unique scent that will activate the brain's center of emotion and memory (the limbic system) in a different way. Some essential oils may uplift the spirits, others help you release negative thoughts and habits. They can be your key to a more fulfilling and balanced emotional life.

You can use the following oils and blends for diffusion, soothing baths, massage, inhalation, or topical application to help you rediscover peace, balance, and joy:

- Joy™
- Lavender
- Orange
- Peace & Calming®
- Peppermint
- Jasmine

IMPROVE YOUR PHYSICAL WELLNESS

Life gets busier and more chaotic each day, and your lifestyle doesn't always create an ideal opportunity to maintain physical wellness. Poor diet, lack of exercise, and being pummeled by environmental toxins can leave the body unbalanced. From cleansing and weight management to supporting all of the systems in your body, essential oils and essential oil-infused supplements, can provide the solutions you need.

Feel alive and refreshed every day with nutrients, powerful antioxidants, and pure essential oils found in these products:

- **NingXia Red®**
- **Life 9™**
- **Slique® Tea**
- **OmegaGize3®**
- **Longevity™**

CLEANSE YOUR HOME AND SURROUNDINGS

You don't have to use harsh chemicals to clean your home. You can polish countertops, remove sticky messes, repel bugs, and clean dirty areas with gentle and effective power of essential oils and Thieves® products.

There are convenient and non-chemical options for cleaning your home, without chemicals, leaving only pleasant scents and a healthy environment. You can replace the cleansers with these versatile products:

- **Lemon**
- **Purification®**
- **Thyme**
- **Lemongrass**
- **Thieves® Household Cleaner**

REFINE YOUR SKIN

Rediscover your natural glow and purge chemicals from your beauty routine. Essential oils can help soothe tension, support healthy cell growth, promote clear complexion, soften signs of aging, and nurture healthy hair. Here are some suggestions:

- **ART® Renewal Serum**
- **Lavender**
- **Lavender Volume Shampoo/Conditioner**
- **Frankincense**
- **Copaiba Vanilla Shampoo/Conditioner**
- **Boswellia Wrinkle Cream™**

PROMOTE SPIRITUAL AWARENESS

Incense and essential oils from plants have always had a starring role in religious and spiritual ceremonies, helping those involved to transcend the trivial and connect with something larger than themselves.

To enhance your spiritual experience, dilute and apply meditative, empowering essential oils directly to wrists, feet, and behind the ears, or diffuse in a quiet area. Popular oils and blends for spiritual focus include:

- · **Sacred Frankincense™**
- · **White Angelica™**
- · **Egyptian Gold™**
- · **Inspiration™**
- · **The Gift™**

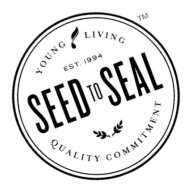

COMMONLY USED COLLECTIONS

Everyday Oils™ Collection

Every day we touch, taste, and inhale harmful chemicals and toxins. Synthetic ingredients are in nearly every item in the home, from cleaning solutions and personal care products to food additives. These oils work as natural, chemical-free alternatives for items you use every day.

- Frankincense *(boswcllia carteri)*
- Lavender *(lavandula angustifolia)*
- Lemon Vitality™ *(citrus limon)*
- Tea Tree *(melaleuca alternifolia)*
- Peppermint Vitality™ *(mentha piperita)*
- Joy™
- Purification®
- PanAway®
- Thieves® Vitality™
- Stress Away™

Premium Starter Kit Essential Oils - 12 Oils

- Lavender
- Lemon Vitality™
- Frankincense
- Raven™
- DiGize™ Vitality™
- Stress Away™
- Peppermint Vitality™
- Valor®
- Thieves® Vitality™
- Citrus Fresh™ Vitality™
- PanAway®
- Peace & Calming®

Raindrop Technique® - 9 Essential Oils

Raindrop Technique® combines aromatherapy with the techniques of Vita Flex and massage in the application of essential oils to various areas of the body.

- Thyme
- Basil
- Peppermint
- Oregano
- Wintergreen
- Cypress
- Marjoram
- Valor®
- Aroma Siez™

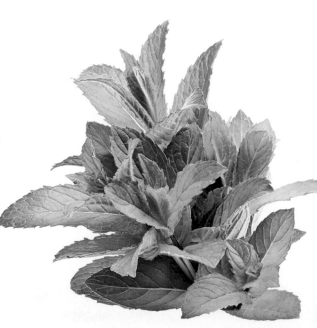

SINGLE OILS

Experience singular notes of pure bliss. These powerful essential oils bring out the very best in you, each and every day.

Angelica (angelica archangelica)
Soothing qualities, relax nerves and muscles, calms anxiety, restores happy memories, brings peaceful sleep, digestive support

Balsam Fir, Idaho (abies balsamea)
Emotional balance, muscular aches and pains, soothes and rejuvenates body and mind

Basil (ocimum basilicum)
Mental clarity, alertness, balancing, can refresh the mind, restores mental alertness, may sharpen sense of smell, useful for fatigued or aching muscles

Bergamot (citrus bergamia)
Confidence, calming, female hormonal support, fresh sweet citrus scent, enhance mood, used for oily and troubled skin

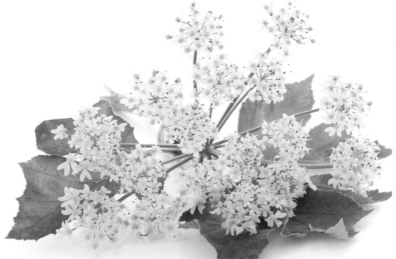

Black Pepper (piper nigrum)
Energizing, endurance, comforting and energizing, used topically for soothing muscle discomfort, enhance flavor of foods

Blue Cypress (callitris intratropica)
Supports body's natural response to irritation and injury, aids normal breathing

Blue Tansy (tanacetum annum)
Relaxation, sweet herbaceous aroma

Cardamom (elettaria cardamomum)
Protects the stomach, invigorates the mind, alleviates mental fatigue

Carrot Seed (daucus carota)
Digestive support, joint support

Cedarwood (cedrus atlantica)
Balancing, relaxing, mental focus, useful for oily skin, soothing during massage

Celery Seed (apium graveolens)
Liver support, digestive support, physical discomfort

Cinnamon Bark (cinnamomum verum)
Immune system support, promote healthy cardiovascular and immune function, acts as an antiseptic, dilute and use for massage

Cistus (cistus ladanifer)
Relaxing and elevating, calming, uplifting, helpful for meditating and counseling

Citronella (cymbopogon nardus)
Respiratory support, insect repellent, relaxing, can delay food spoilage due to fungus

Clary Sage (salvia sclarea)
Stress relief, female hormonal support, relaxing, supports normal healthy attitude during PMS

Clove (syzygium aromaticum)
Antioxidant support, digestive support, physical discomfort, stimulating and revitalizing

Copaiba (copaifera reticulata)
Physical discomfort, aids digestion, and supports body's natural response to injury or irritation

Coriander (coriandrum sativum)
Pancreatic support, digestive support, soothing and calming properties, supports healthy digestive and circulatory system functions

Cypress (cupressus sempervirens)
Grounding, restores feelings of security and stability, beneficial for oily or troubled skin

Dill (anethum graveolens)
Flavorant, calming, digestive support, balancing, stimulating, and revitalizing

Dorado Azul
Topical and aromatic use

Elemi (canarium luzonicum)
Grounding, traditionally used for skin, reduce look of fine lines and wrinkles, soothing muscles

Eucalyptus Blue
Calming, topical, and aromatic use

Eucalyptus Globulus (eucalyptus globulus)
Key ingredient in many mouth rinses, applied topically in respiratory system, soothe muscles after exercise

Eucalyptus Radiata (eucalyptus radiata)
Purifying, cleansing, relatively gentle and non-irritating, suitable for topical use

Fennel (foeniculum vulgare)
Women's health, digestive support, stimulating to circulatory, glandular, respiratory and digestive systems, support during menstrual cycle

Frankincense (boswellia carteri)
Immune support, skin health, spiritual grounding, stimulating and elevating to the mind, help focus the mind, overcome stress and despair

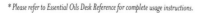

Galbanum (ferula gummosa)
Spiritual grounding, supports systems including immune, digestive, respiratory, and circulatory

Geranium (pelargonium graveolens)
Respiratory support, liver support, women's health, excellent for the skin, helps release negative memories, supports circulatory and nervous systems

German Chaomile (matricaria recutita)
Liver and gallbladder support, relaxing, supports natural response to irritation and injury

Ginger (zingiber officinale)
Muscle tension, digestive support, stamina

Goldenrod (solidago canadensis)
Libido, circulatory support, supports urinary tract, liver function

Grapefruit (citrus paradisi)
Energizing and uplifting, nourishes the skin

Helichrysum (helichrysum italicum)
Circulatory support, muscle tension, restorative properties, supports nervous system, skin, liver

Hinoki (chamaecyparis obtusa)
Spiritual awareness, energizes and uplifts the mind, calming and relaxing during agitation

Hong Kuai (chamaecyparis formosensis)
Supports deep sense of relaxation, spiritual awareness, abundant aromatic nature

Hyssop (hyssopus officinalis)
Slightly sweet, purifying

Idaho Blue Spruce
Muscle tension, emotional release

Idaho Tansy (tanacetum vulgare)
Stimulates positive attitude and general feeling of well-being, soothing to the skin

Jasmine (jasminum officinale)
Relaxes, soothes, uplifts and enhances self-confidence, used to balance feminine energy

Juniper (Juniperus osteosperma and scopulorum)
Cleansing effect on the mind, spirit and body, detoxifier and cleanser, beneficial to the skin

Laurus Nobilis (laurus nobilis)
Respiratory support, grounding, calming

Lavender (lavandula angustifolia)
Skin irritations, balancing, relaxing, soothing and refreshing, good for relaxing and winding down before bedtime, boosts stamina

* Please refer to Essential Oils Desk Reference for complete usage instructions.

Ledum (ledum groenlandicum)
Cleansing, provides well-being, believed to harmonize and balance the body's daily needs

Lemon (citrus limon)
Energizing, circulatory support, cleansing, beneficial to the skin, enhance flavor of foods, supports nervous and sympathetic systems

Lemon Myrtle (backhousia citriodora)
Mental clarity, immune support, purifying, boosts natural defenses, can act as cleansing agent to purify household surfaces

Lemongrass (cymbopogon flexuosus)
Purifying, digestive support, rejuvenating, improves mental clarity, supports circulatory system

Lime (citrus latifolia)
Invigorating and stimulating effect, may help mental clarity and encourage creativity, supports healthy immune system

Marjoram (origanum majorana)
Muscle tension, calming, relaxing, occasional simple nervous tension

Melaleuca (alternifolia)
Cleansing, supports immune system and benefits the skin

Melaleuca Quinquenervia (niaouli)
Supports skin health

Melissa (melissa officinalis)
Strengthening and revitalizing, soothing and calming, may benefit the skin, supports immune system

Mountain Savory (satureja montana)
General tonic for the body, provides support for the immune, nervous, and circulatory systems

Myrrh (commipihora myrrha)
Spiritual awareness, skin health, antioxidant support, revitalizing and uplifting, widely used in oral hygiene products

Myrtle (Myrtus communis)
Respiratory support, thyroid support, emotional balance, supportive system for skin and hair

Neroli (citrus aurantium)
Mental clarity, emotional balance, believed to have healing properties

Nutmeg (myristica fragrans)
Energizing, helps boost energy, supports nervous and endocrine systems

Ocotea (ocotea quixos)
Purifying, digestive support, satiety, helps aid body's natural response to irritation and injury

Orange (citrus sinensis)
Cellular support, uplifting, emotional balance, calming influence on the body, aids in maintaining normal cellular regeneration

Oregano (origanum vulgare)
Purifying, contains strong immune enhancing and antioxidant properties, supports respiratory system

Palmarosa (cymbopogon martini)
Cellular support, skin health, balancing

Palo Santo (bursera graveolens)
Spiritual grounding, emotional balance, used to purify and cleanse the spirit of negative energies

Patchouli (pogostemon cablin)
Skin health, emotional release, anti-nausea support, general health support, releases negative emotions

Peppermint (mentha piperita)
Energizing, digestive support, may improve taste and smell when inhaled, may help improve concentration and mental sharpness

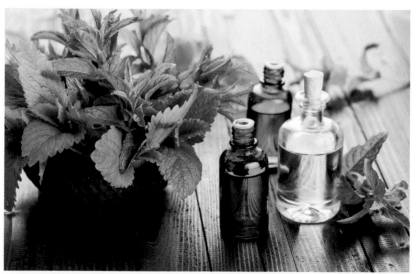

Petitgrain (citrus sinensis)
Skin health, emotional balance, nervous system support, beneficial for skin and hair health

Pine (pinus sylvestris)
Respiratory support, emotional balance, soothes stressed muscles and joints when used in massage

Ravintsara (cinnamomum camphora)
Purifying, meditation, similar to eucalyptus but softer, spicy

Roman Chamomile (chamaemelum nobile)
Skin health, relaxing, muscle tension, gentle effects especially valuable for restless children, beneficial when added to massage oil

Rose (rosa damascena)
Skin health, emotional release, energy balance, simulating and uplifting properties

Rosemary (rosmarinus officinalis CT cineol)
Mental clarity, liver support, may help restore mental alertness when experiencing fatigue

Royal Hawaiian Sandalwood (santalum paniculatum)
Uplifting, relaxing, valued in skin care, moisturizing and normalizing properties

Sacred Frankincense™ (boswellia sacra)
Ideal for those wishing to take their spiritual journey and meditation experiences to higher level

* Please refer to Essential Oils Desk Reference for complete usage instructions.

-25-

Sage (salvia officinalis)
Mental balance, skin health, women's health, supports respiratory, reproductive, and nervous systems

Spearmint (nentha spicata)
Emotional release, digestive support, respiratory health, leads to sense of balance and well-being

Spikenard (nardostachys jatamansi)
Relaxing, soothing for the skin

Lavender (lavandula angustifolia)
Skin irritations, balancing, relaxing, soothes and cleanses minor cuts, bruises and skin irritations

Tangerine (citrus reticulata)
Antioxidant support, digestive support, satiety, uplifts the spirit and brings sense of security

Tarragon (artemisia dracunculus)
Digestive support, adds special touch when used as a spice in recipes

Thyme (thymus vulgaris)
Immune support, purifying, cleansing, supports immune, respiratory, digestive, nervous, and other body systems

Tsuga (tsuga canadensis)
Spiritual balance, used to make poultices

Valerian (valeriana officinalis)
Calming, sleep support, emotional balance, believed to have relaxing properties, calming and restorative effects on nervous system

Vetiver (vetiveria zizanoides)
Emotional grounding, sleep support, relaxing, supports coping with stress and recovering from emotional trauma and shock

Wintergreen (gaultheria procumbens)
Flavors numerous products, beneficial in massage and soothing head tension and muscles after exercising

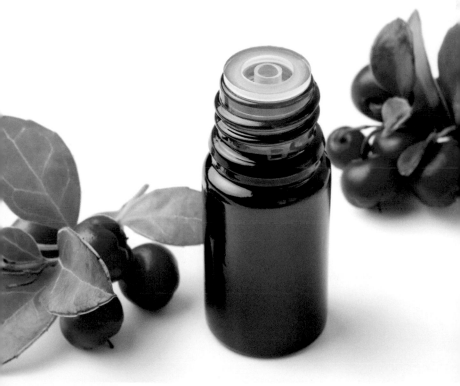

* Please refer to Essential Oils Desk Reference for complete usage instructions.

-27-

Xiang Mao (cymbopogon citratus)
Spiritual awareness, calming, relaxing, and cleansing

Ylang Ylang (cananga odorata)
Circulatory support, emotional balance
Whether you need to boost your brainpower or de-stress and unwind,
we've got specially formulated essential oil blends that are just right for you.
Invigorate your senses and transform your day.

BLENDED OILS

*Transform your day and awaken
your senses with formulated
essential oil blends designed
to meet your daily needs.*

COMMONLY USED BLENDED OILS

BLENDED OILS

Abundance™
Emotional support, energizing, attracts prosperity
Abundance™ opens us to a wealth of possibilities

Acceptance™
Acceptance™, self-worth, stimulates the mind, helps overcome
procrastination and denial

Aroma Life™
Combines Ylang Ylang with known powerhouses Cypress, Helichrysum, and
Marjoram

Aroma Siez™
Well suited for use after exercise, combined with massage oil, provides
soothing comfort for head, neck, and tired feet

AromaEase™
Soothes occasional stress, helps support healthy energy flow and vitality

Australian Blue™
Uplifts and inspires the mind and heart, calming and stabilizing

Awaken™
Helps awaken potential, supports making necessary changes to manifest
dreams and goals

Brain Power™
Use it to clarify thought and develop focus

Build Your Dream™
Includes significant oils that highlight a lifetime journey of helping individuals discover profound and lasting transformations, improve their health, and change lives around the world

Christmas Spirit™
Purify and energy balance, helps tap into happiness, joy and security associated with the holiday season

Citrus Fresh™
Mental clarity, energizing, purifying, supports immune system, and overall health

Clarity™
Promotes mental sharpness, restores mental alertness or wakefulness when you're fatigued or drowsy

Common Sense™
Enhances rational decision making abilities, leading to increased wellness, purpose, and abundance

DiGize™
Helps support a healthy digestive system

Dragon Time™
Perfect choice for women's emotions during special times and needs Promotes balance and normal healthy emotions

Dream Catcher™
Spiritual awareness, enhances ability to hold onto dreams, protects against negative dreams that may cloud vision

Please refer to Essential Oils Desk Reference for complete usage instructions.

Egyptian Gold™
Spiritual awareness, immune support, enhances moments of devotion and reverence

En-R-Gee™
Helps restore mental alertness, boosts energy

Endoflex™
Endocrine support, female hormonal support

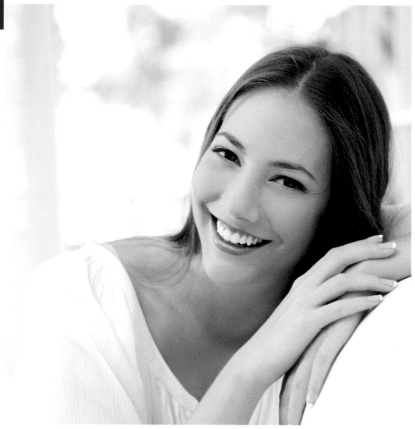

Envision™
Emotional release, renew focus, stimulates creativity and resourcefulness, encourages renewed faith in the future

Evergreen Essence™
Refreshes the senses, get back to nature by combining aromatic scents of pine, cedar, and spruce trees

Exodus II™
Cleansing, timeless blend of oils

Forgiveness™
Emotional support, emotional release, energy balance, soothing and uplifting oils that may enhance the ability to release hurtful memories and move beyond emotional barriers

GLF™
Blend of powerful oils including Helichrysum, Spearmint, and Celery Seed, applied topically over the liver and on Vita Flex points on the feet

Gathering™
Spiritual grounding, emotional balance, helps overcome chaotic energy, helps gather emotional and spiritual forces to achieve greater unity of purpose

Gentle Baby™
Calming, relaxing, designed especially for mothers and babies, helps calm emotions during pregnancy and is useful for quieting little ones, soothing to tender skin

BLENDED OILS

Gratitude™

Spiritual grounding, emotional balance, designed to elevate the spirit, calm emotions, fosters grateful attitude

Grounding™

Mental clarity, stress relief, emotional balance, may aid in coping with reality in a positive way

Harmony™

Stress relief, energy balance, promotes physical and emotional well-being by bringing harmonic balance to the energy centers of the body

Highest Potential™

Confidence, emotional balance, designed to increase your capacity to achieve your highest potential, soothes, and harmonizes

Hope™

Emotional grounding, emotional strength, designed to uplift and balance emotions, may help to overcome severe dark thoughts

Humility™

Spiritual awareness, emotional balance, emotional strength, may bring balance to your heart and mind, promoting emotional healing

ImmuPower™

Creates a fragrant and protective haven while increasing positive energy

Inner Child™

Emotional release, emotional balance, opens pathways to connect with the inner self that may have been misused or abused in childhood

Inspiration™
Spiritual awareness, calming, enhancing spirituality, prayer, meditation, and inner awareness, creates aromatic sanctuary

Into the Future™
Confidence, decision-making, emotional release, fosters feelings of determination, leaving the past behind so you can move forward, enhances enjoyment of challenges

Joy™
Emotional balance, uplifting, creates magnetic energy and brings joy to the heart, may exude an irresistible fragrance inspiring togetherness

Juva Cleanse®
Supports normal liver function, balancing

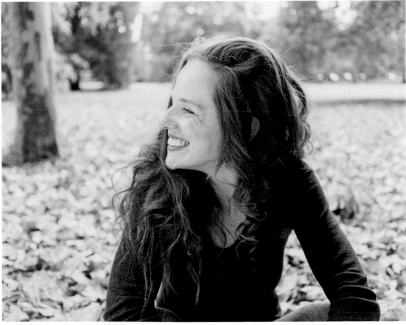

BLENDED OILS

Juva Flex™
Liver support, digestive support, may also support healthy cell function

Lady Sclareol™
Designed as an exquisite fragrance, creating a beguiling and alluring perfume

BLENDED OILS

Live with Passion™
Helps revive the zest for life, improves internal energy, formulated specifically to help recover an optimistic attitude

Longevity™
Antioxidant support, help neutralizes free radicals and lessen the daily oxidative damage

M-Grain™
Calming, promotes sense of well-being particularly in the head and neck area

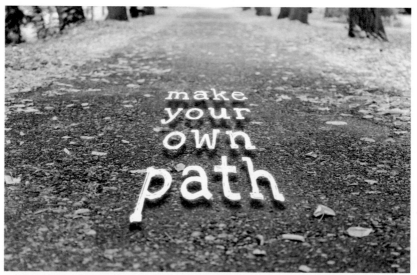

Magnify Your Purpose™
Mental clarity, motivation, stimulates desire, focus and motivation, helps foster positive attitude

Melrose™
Skin health, cleansing, provides a protective barrier against skin challenges, can help dispel odors

Mister™
Emotional balance, helps promote greater inner body balance, may be soothing while stressed, recommended for males 30 years and over

Motivation™
Positive energy, emotional release, motivation, may help enable one to surmount fear and procrastination, while stimulating feelings of action and accomplishment

PanAway®
Often used for massage and soothing skin, while providing comfort to muscles after exercise

Peace & Calming®
Gentle fragrant blend, helps calm tension and uplift the spirit, promotes relaxation and a deep sense of peace

Present Time™
Empowerment, emotional release, may heighten the sense of being "in the moment"

Purification®
Cleansing, used directly on skin to clean and soothe, helps purify air when diffused

BLENDED OILS

* Please refer to Essential Oils Desk Reference for complete usage instructions.

R.C.™
May be invigorating when applied to chest and throat, wonderful blend to diffuse during winter

Raven™
Combination of soothing oils, provides comfort when applied topically to chest and throat or when diffused

Release™
Emotional release and balance, stimulates sense of peace and emotional well-being, may facilitate the ability to release anger and frustration

Relieve It™
Deeply relaxing, soothing and comforting to muscles and joints following exercise

RutaVaLa™
Stress relieving, relaxing, helps ease tension

SARA™
Emotional release, emotional healing, relaxing, may help soothe deep emotional wounds

Sacred Mountain™
Empowerment, emotional balance, emotional strength, promotes feelings of strength, grounding, and protection

SclarEssence™
Female hormonal support, energy balance, women's health, calming action for an extraordinary dietary supplement

Sensation™
Romantic emotions, skin health, extremely uplifting and refreshing

Slique™ Essence
Weight management support, satiety, supports healthy weight management goals, may help with hunger and digestion

Stress Away™
Designed to combat normal everyday stresses, reduce mental rigidity, and restore equilibrium

BLENDED OILS

Surrender™
Emotional release and balance, helps quiet troubled hearts so that negative emotions can be released, return feelings of equilibrium

The Gift™
Immune support, calming effects

Thieves®
Immune support, purifying, tested for its cleansing abilities, supports good health

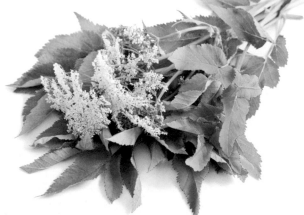

* Please refer to Essential Oil Desk Reference for complete usage instructions.

Three (3) Wise Men™
Spiritual awareness, promotes feelings of reverence, formulated to open the subconscious

Transformation™
Emotional release, empowers you to replace negative beliefs with uplifting thoughts, changing your overall attitude, emotions, and behavior

Trauma Life™
Stress relief, emotional release, formulated to help release buried emotional trauma resulting from accidents, neglect, death, assault or abuse

White Angelica™
Spiritual awareness, energy balance, encourages feelings of protection and security to bring about sense of strength and endurance

YL Oola® Balance™
Designed to align and balance your center, giving you an increase in concentration with a positive outlook. The balance between mind and body, increasing the ability to focus on passions, behaviors, and health.

YL Oola® Grow™
Designed to help you reach unlimited potential and growth in many aspects of life. Gives you courage to focus on the task at hand and help move forward with positive advancements and progression.

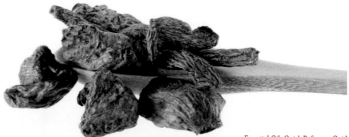

VITALITY OILS

The Vitality™ line of essential oils provides a variety of options to share your favorite oils in delicious and nutritious ways – celebrate food, family, and life!

Basil Vitality™

Basil Vitality™ easily pairs with savory foods, but can also complement any meal with its sweet, slightly peppery flavor. Add a few drops to your soups, sauces, and meats, or pair with juice and melons for a lighter treat.

Bergamot Vitality™

Best paired with summer dishes, Bergamot Vitality™ has a fresh, tart, citrus flavor. It has a distinct sour orange/lemon flavor and can easily be added to sugarless baked goods to brighten the flavor.

Black Pepper Vitality™

This blend is easily used in rubs and marinades for meat and seafood, as well as in dressings for salads. It has the most common and potent flavor of the peppercorn family.

Cardamom Vitality™

Cardamom is often used to enhance the flavor of hot drinks and is one of the world's favorite cooking spices. It is often used in both sweet and savory dishes, including baked goods.

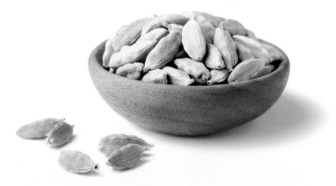

VITALITY

Carrot Seed Vitality™

Use a few drops of Carrot Seed Vitality™ in salad dressings for a richer flavor. Enhance the earthy flavor of roasted vegetables or rice, by adding a drop of oil before serving.

Celery Seed Vitality™

Celery Seed Vitality™ can quickly bring a pleasant taste and aroma to brines and pickling juices. The flavor is often referred to as grassy and earthy, but can also enhance the flavor of chicken, coleslaw, and dressings.

Cinnamon Bark Vitality™

Cinnamon Bark provides a potent flavor known for its unique and spicy notes. It can be used as a dietary supplement and adds warm hints to many culinary treats.

Citrus Fresh™ Vitality™

This blend offers a unique combination of Orange, Mandarin, Tangerine, Grapefruit, and Lemon oils with a burst of Spearmint flavor. It is ideal for adding to juices and water to add a bit of freshness.

Clove Vitality™

This has been distilled from the same spicy cloves that have been enjoyed in kitchens for generations. Use in both sweet and savory dishes. Clove Vitality™ may also support overall wellness.

Copaiba Vitality™

This unique oil offers a sweet aroma and has a pleasant, complex taste that can promote wellness. Add a drop or two to your tea to complement a healthy diet.

VITALITY

Coriander Vitality™

Coriander shares origins with cilantro making it ideal in both Latin and Eastern dishes. Mix in with your favorite marinades and dressings to add a layer of flavor.

DiGize™ Vitality™

DiGize is a great blend of Ginger, Peppermint, Juniper, Tarragon, Fennel, Lemongrass, Anise, and Patchouli oils and offers a fresh taste. It is even sweeter when combined with honey.

Dill Vitality™

This essential oil provides a fresh flavor that is a great substitute for dried dill in dressings and dips. It can also be added as a flavorful ingredient to soups and stews. Dill Vitality™ is a key flavor in many Russian, Mediterranean, Asian, and many other cuisines.

EndoFlex™ Vitality™

EndoFlex™ has a base of sesame seed oil and can offer wellness support. It can be added to water, juice or warm tea as well. When added to NingXia Zyng™ it can give you a jump-start to your day.

Fennel Vitality™

Fennel Vitality™ has a distinct licorice flavor and may be added to sauces, soups, and more for an extra rich and savory taste. Add a drop or two to a warm glass of water after meals.

Frankincense Vitality™

This can be used to enhance the taste and aroma of foods with its sweet and woodsy flavor. The benefits of Frankincense Vitality™ include supporting well-being and cellular health. Add to juice or water or a shot of NingXia Red®.

GLF™ Vitality™

Use GLF™ Vitality™ as a dietary supplement. It includes Grapefruit, Ledum, Helichrysum, Hyssop, Celery Seed, and Spearmint and can be added to a daily green smoothie or glass of juice. It has amazing intestinal cleansing benefits.

German Chamomile Vitality™

This is steamed from German Chamomile flowers and has a delicate apple taste. It may be used in salad dressings or tea and can bc used to aid digestive health.

Ginger Vitality™

Ginger can be used in the kitchen as a flavorful additive as well as a dietary supplement. It is a distinct and versatile oil and may be included in sweet or savory dishes. You may also enjoy adding a drop to your tea.

Grapefruit Vitality™

Grapefruit is well known for a strong citrus scent and a delicious, tart flavor. It can be used to support weight management programs when paired with a healthy diet and exercise. Add to drinks to add a hint of citrus to many culinary recipes.

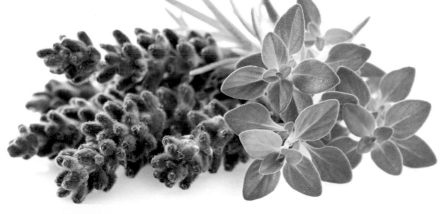

VITALITY

Jade Lemon Vitality™

Jade Lemon Vitality™ offers a great lemon-lime taste to any beverage. When added to other culinary delights including baked treats, it can add a bright citrusy flavor and invigorate the senses. Add to yogurt or tea.

Juva Cleanse® Vitality™

Use this along with fiber rich foods to promote a healthy digestive system. Add a drop or two to water and enjoy the cleansing benefits. To enhance wellness, take with JuvaTone™ daily between meals.

JuvaFlex™ Vitality™

Take as a dietary supplement to help support overall wellness. May be combined with JuvaTone™ daily. Add to your favorite green shake to enjoy powerful antioxidant benefits.

Laurus Nobilis Vitality™

May be used in hearty stews and soups to provide a distinct bay leaf flavoring. May also be used in marinades, sauces, and pickles. Add drops to glass of hot water to enjoy before meals. Use as a dietary supplement.

Lavender Vitality™

Although known for adding a great flavor to sweeter dishes, Lavender Vitality™ may also be added savory dishes as well. Start small when using in recipes to avoid overwhelming the flavor. Can be used when making homemade fruit jams as well.

Lemon Vitality™

Lemon Vitality™ can add a bright flavor to many dishes. It can be very versatile and may be used in both sweet and savory dishes, including fish and chicken as well as pastries and cakes. Can be used as a convenient substitute for fresh zest or juice. Add a drop to cold water as a fresh start to your day.

Lemongrass Vitality™

The bright and lemony scent can support wellness when added to drinks or used as a supplement. It has a delicate citrus flavor when added to Asian recipes. Add a couple of drops to water or tea.

Lime Vitality™

Lime Vitality™ will add a zesty citrusy flavor to any recipe. Elevate your cooking with a couple of drops to any food or drink. Enjoy a year round kick of summer by adding this concentrated and versatile oil.

Longevity™ Vitality™

This powerful combination includes Thyme, Orange, Clove, and Frankincense and can be included in your healthy wellness regimen. This is perfect for those getting up in their senior years and can help support a healthy immune system.

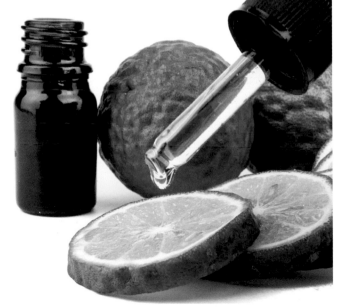

* Please refer to Essential Oils Desk Reference for complete usage instructions.

-47-

Marjoram Vitality™

Marjoram can be found in savory dishes and has a flavor similar to oregano; it perfectly complements Italian cuisine and other delicate foods like fish and vegetables. Add a drop or two to replace fresh Marjoram in any recipe.

Mountain Savory Vitality™

May be used as a culinary herb and has a strong, warm flavor that is similar to oregano. It can be a useful addition to your pantry and may be used as a dietary supplement. The spicy herbaceous flavor can enhance the flavors of meats and beans.

Nutmeg Vitality™

Nutmeg offers a warm and nostalgic taste to spice cakes and teas. This powerful and versatile oil can be added to winter produce like squash and pumpkin as well as holiday baked goods.

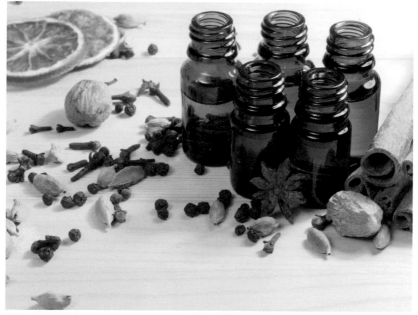

Orange Vitality™

Orange offers a clean and refreshing scent and can be used as a part of a wellness plan. May be used in cooking to brighten up dishes with a bright citrus flavor. Add it to baked goods to enhance an acidic taste and increase the contrast with the sweet flavor.

Oregano Vitality™

Oregano Vitality™ can help support a healthy lifestyle when taken as a dietary supplement. It is an easy way to add flavor to savory dishes and enhances the distinctive, pungent flavor of Mediterranean and Mexican cuisines.

Peppermint Vitality™

This oil offers a bright and cool flavor with benefits of gastrointestinal comfort and digestive support as well. May be added to meals and water to support exercise performance. Add to teas and your baking recipes as well.

VITALITY

Rosemary Vitality™

Rosemary is used as a flavorful additive in many cuisines, especially Italian dishes. It is perfect for savory recipes. Add to tomato sauce and other pasta and breads for an authentic robust flavor.

Sage Vitality™

Although most commonly used with holiday feasts, this is a great year-round seasoning. Enhance the flavor of seafood, vegetables, and many savory breads. May be taken as a dietary supplement to help support a healthy digestive system.

SclarEssence™ Vitality™

Most often used with women's wellness regimens and includes Clary Sage, Peppermint, Sage, and Fennel. Add to a warm cup of tea or glass of water. May be combined with Master Formula™.

Spearmint Vitality™

Spearmint has the unique mint flavor that supports normal digestion. Can be added to food for a cooling effect. Add to a glass of fruit infused water or tea to promote healthy hydration.

Tangerine Vitality™

This can add citrusy notes to savory dishes and desserts and can bring a bright and tangy addition to your kitchen. May be used as a part of a daily dietary supplement. A drop or two added to marinades can add a sweet kick. Enjoy drinking more water by adding a few drops to each sparkling glass.

Tarragon Vitality™

Tarragon is often used in French cooking and offers a distinctly strong herbaceous flavor to your favorite dishes. It pairs well with fish, meat, and soups. It is a perfect complement to savory dishes and sauces. May be used as a dietary supplement.

Thieves® Vitality™

Add a drop or two into a capsule as a part of a dietary supplement. Can also be swirled into your juice or morning coffee to give you a flavorful boost. May be added to oatmeal, granola or other cereal to enhance your morning breakfast routine.

Thyme Vitality™

A long time classic herb that can be used in place of dried Thyme in all of your favorite dishes. It is a great supplement to your healthy lifestyle. Place in your next pasta or poultry dish to add a layer of flavor. Use a few drops in your marinades to infuse meats and vegetables with an herbal richness.

KIDS

Our KidScents® proprietary blends and other products are safe alternatives to products for children commonly found in the market today. You'll love our kid-focused essential oil blends and other products.

KidScents® Body Care for Children
Our KidScents® proprietary blends and other products are safe alternatives to products for children commonly found in the market today. You'll love our kid-focused essential oil blends and other products.

KidScents® Bath Gel
KidScents® Bath Gel is a safe and gentle formula with a neutral pH balance perfect for young skin. It contains no mineral oils, synthetic perfumes, artificial colorings, or toxic ingredients.

<u>Ingredients:</u> water, decyl glucoside, glycerin, sorbitol, dimethyl sulfone (MSM), Roman chamomile flower extract, aloe vera leaf juice, panthenol, tocopheryl acetate (vitamin E), PG-hydroxyethylcellulose cocodimonium chloride, coneflower extract, grape seed extract, soap bark extract, soapwort extract, kiwi seed oil, jojoba seed oil, grapefruit seed extract

<u>Essential Oils:</u> Cedarwood, Geranium

<u>Directions:</u> Apply a small amount of KidScents® Bath Gel to washcloth or directly to the skin. Rub gently, then rinse.

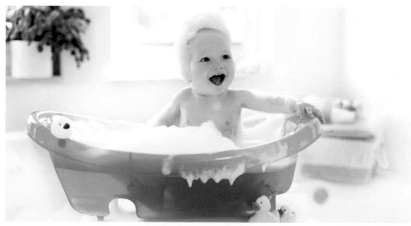

KidScents® Lotion

KidScents® Lotion is safe, gentle, and pH neutral, ideal for young skin. It contains no mineral oils, synthetic perfumes, artificial colorings, or toxic ingredients.

Ingredients: water, dimethyl sulfone (MSM), glyceryl stearate, stearic acid, glycerin, grape seed extract, sodium hyaluronate, sorbitol, rose hip seed oil, shea butter, mango seed butter, wheat germ oil, kukui seed oil, lecithin, safflower seed oil, apricot kernel oil, sweet almond oil, vitamin E (tocopheryl acetate), vitamin A (retinyl palmitate), jojoba seed oil, sesame seed oil, marigold flower extract, matricaria (Roman chamomile) flower extract, green tea leaf extract, St. John's wort extract, algae extract, aloe vera leaf juice, ascorbic acid, ginkgo biloba leaf extract

Essential Oils: Cedarwood, Coriander, Geranium, Western Red Cedar, Bergamot (Furocoumarin-free), Ylang Ylang

Directions: Apply liberally to skin as needed.

KidScents® Shampoo

KidScents® Shampoo contains the finest natural ingredients for gently cleansing children's delicate hair. A mild formula designed to provide the perfect pH balance for children's hair, it contains no mineral oils, synthetic perfumes, artificial colorings, or toxic ingredients.

Ingredients: water, decyl glucoside, dimethyl sulfone (MSM), Roman chamomile flower extract, aloe vera leaf juice, vitamin B5 (panthenol), vitamin E (tocopheryl acetate), babassu seed oil, coneflower extract, kiwi seed oil, jojoba seed oil, grape seed extract

Essential Oils: Tangerine, Lemon

Directions: Apply a small amount to hair. Lather, then rinse.

KIDS

KidScents® Slique® Toothpaste

KidScents® Slique® Toothpaste is a safe, natural alternative to commercial brands of toothpaste. Formulated with Slique™ Essence and Thieves® essential oil blends, this toothpaste gently cleans teeth and tastes great without synthetic dyes or flavors. Slique™ Essence is antibacterial, antifungal, a lipid regulator, and a glucose regulator. Thieves® is antiseptic, antimicrobial, and combats plaque-causing micro-organisms.

Ingredients: water, calcium carbonate, coconut oil, baking soda (sodium bicarbonate), vegetable glycerin, xylitol, xanthan gum, stevia leaf extract, lecithin

Essential Oils: Grapefruit, Tangerine, Spearmint, Lemon, Ocotea, Clove, Cinnamon Bark, Eucalyptus Radiata, Rosemary

Directions: Brush teeth thoroughly after meals or at least 2 times daily.

KidScents® Tender Tush™

KidScents® Tender Tush™ is a gentle ointment designed to protect and nourish young skin and promote healing. This ointment soothes dry, chapped skin and offers protection for delicate skin. It is also great for expectant mothers who are concerned about having stretch marks.

Ingredients: coconut oil, cocoa seed butter, olive fruit oil, sweet almond oil, beeswax, wheat germ oil

Essential Oils: Royal Hawaiian Sandalwood, Coriander, Roman Chamomile, Lavender, Frankincense, Bergamot (furocoumarin-free), Cistus, Ylang Ylang, Geranium

Directions: Apply liberally to diaper area as often as needed to help soothe diaper rash, redness, or irritation.

KIDS

KidScents® Nutritional Support for Children

KidScents® MightyPro™

Support is here for children's digestive and immune health with a delicious wolfberry punch flavor. This KidScents® supplement delivers the synergistic power of pre- and probiotics with over 8 billion active, live cultures of the friendly bacteria needed for optimal health.

Ingredients: fructooligosaccharides, lactobacillus paracasei Lpc-37, lactobacillus acidophilus LA-14, goji fruit powder

Other Ingredients: xylitol, erythritol, natural fruit punch flavor, citric acid

Directions: For children 2 years and above, empty entire content of 1 packet into mouth and allow it to dissolve. Take 1 packet daily with food to provide optimal conditions for healthy gut bacteria. Can be taken straight or combined with applesauce, yogurt, or other food or beverage. Do not add to warm or hot food or beverage.

Caution: *Keep out of reach of children. Do not exceed recommended dosage. Adults may also take this supplement. If pregnant or nursing, taking medication, or having a medical condition, consult a health care professional prior to use.*

KIDS

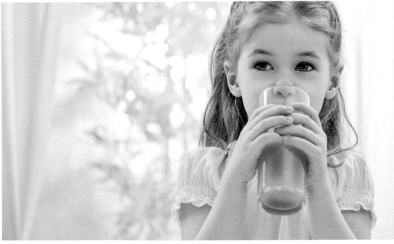

KidScents® MightyVites™

KidScents® MightyVites™ is a whole-food multinutrient that contains super fruits, plants, and vegetables that deliver the full spectrum of vitamins, minerals, antioxidants, and phytonutrients, specifically designed for children's developing bodies. Children's diets often need a bridge between what they are eating and what they should be eating. To fuel growth and normal activity levels, a child's diet must provide plenty of vitamins and minerals as well as support stores of nutrients in preparation for the accelerated growth spurts of the teenage years.

Ingredients: vitamin A, vitamin C (as ascorbic acid from orange), vitamin D (as cholecalciferol), vitamin E (as d-alpha tocopheryl acid succinate), thiamine (vitamin B1 as thiamine mononitrate), riboflavin (vitamin B2), niacin (as niacinamide), vitamin B6 (from organic food blends), folate (from organic food blend), vitamin B12 (methylcobalamin), and more

MightyVites™ Wild Berry Blend: Orgen-Kid: [curry leaf extract, guava fruit extract, lemon peel extract, sesbania leaf extract, amala fruit extract, holy basil aerial parts extract, annatto seed extract, beet root juice powder, orange fruit juice powder, strawberry fruit juice powder, wolfberry fruit powder, citrus flavonoids (from tangerine peel), barley grass leaf powder, broccoli sprout powder]

Allergen Warning: *Contains an ingredient derived from soy.*

KidScents® MightyZyme™

KidScents® MightyZyme™ is an all-natural, vegetarian, chewable tablet designed to give children added enzyme nutrition to prevent any enzyme depletion, which is a precursor to body dysfunction that can impede growth and brain development. Children today face a world of fast foods and nutritionally depleted foods that are practically devoid of enzymes critical for the proper function of everything from breathing, thinking, circulation, and digestion.

KIDS

MightyZyme™ combines nine different digestive enzymes with several other nutrients to support healthy digestion and relieve occasional symptoms—such as stomach pressure, bloating, gas, pain, and minor cramping—that may occur after eating.

Ingredients: calcium (from calcium carbonate)

Proprietary MightyZyme™ Blend: [lipase, alfalfa leaf powder, amylase, protease 4.5, bromelain, carrot root powder, peptidase, phytase, protease 6.0, protease 3.0, Peppermint oil, cellulase], sorbitol, dextratcs, natural mixed berry flavor, microcrystalline cellulose, magnesium stearate, steric acid, silica, apple juice powder, stevia rebaudiana leaf extract

Essential Oil: Peppermint

Directions: For children age 6 or older: chew 1 tablet 3 times daily prior to or with meals. For children ages 2-6 years of age: chew 1/2 to 1 tablet (crushed if needed and mixed with yogurt or applesauce). Use for relief of occasional symptoms, including fullness, pressure, bloating, stuffed feeling (commonly referred to as gas), pain, and/or minor cramping that may occur after eating.

KIDS

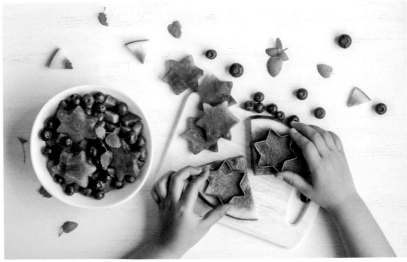

* Please refer to Essential Oils Desk Reference for complete usage instructions.

-57-

KidScents® Oil Collection

The KidScents® Oil Collection includes six oil blends formulated especially for kids to help them through the common ups and downs of childhood.

GeneYus™

Diffuse GeneYus™ to help young minds focus and concentrate on projects.
Ingredients: fractionated coconut oil, Sacred Frankincense™, Blue Cypress, Cedarwood, Idaho Blue Spruce, Palo Santo, Melissa, Northern Lights Black Spruce, almond oil, Bergamot, Myrrh, Vetiver, Geranium, Royal Hawaiian Sandalwood, Ylang Ylang, Hyssop, Rose
Aromatic: Diffuse up to 1 hour 3 times daily.
Topical: Recommended application is for children ages 2-12. To be applied only by a trusted adult or under adult supervision. Apply 2-4 drops directly to desired area. Dilution not required, except for the most sensitive skin. Use as needed.
Caution: *Avoid direct sunlight and UV rays for up to 12 hours after applying product.*

Owie™

Apply Owie™ topically to improve the appearance of your child's skin and help heal wounds.
Ingredients: caprylic/capric glycerides, Idaho Balsam Fir, Tea Tree, Helichrysum, Elemi, Cistus, Hinoki, Clove
Aromatic: Diffuse up to 1 hour 3 times daily.
Topical: Recommended application is for children ages 2-12. To be applied only by a trusted adult or under adult supervision. Apply to desired area as needed. Dilution not required, except for the most sensitive skin.

Sleepylze™

Sleepylze™ calms and relaxes the mind and body prior to bedtime for kids.
Ingredients: caprylic/capric glycerides, Lavender, Geranium, Roman Chamomile, Tangerine, Bergamot, Sacred Frankincense™, Valerian, Rue
Aromatic: Diffuse up to 1 hour 3 times daily.
Topical: Recommended application is for children ages 2-12. To be applied only by a trusted adult or under adult supervision. Apply 2-4 drops directly to desired area. Dilution not required, except for the most sensitive skin. Use as needed. Caution: *Avoid direct sunlight or UV rays for up to 12 hours after applying product.*

SniffleEase™

SniffleEase™ is a refreshing, rejuvenating blend formulated just for kids for when they have congestion.
Ingredients: caprylic/capric glycerides, Eucalyptus Blue, Palo Santo, Lavender, Dorado Azul, Ravintsara, Myrtle, Eucalyptus Globulus, Marjoram, Pine, Eucalyptus Citriodora, Cypress, Eucalyptus Radiata, Northern Lights Black Spruce, Peppermint
Aromatic: Diffuse up to 1 hour 3 times daily.
Topical: Recommended application is for children ages 2-12. To be applied only by a trusted adult or under adult supervision. Apply 2-4 drops directly to desired area. Dilution not required, except for the most sensitive skin. Use as needed.

KIDS

TummyGize™

TummyGize™ is a quieting, relaxing blend that can be applied to little tummies that are upset. It also supports proper digestion.
Ingredients: caprylic/capric glycerides, Spearmint, Peppermint, Tangerine, Fennel, Anise, Ginger, Cardamom
Aromatic: Diffuse up to 1 hour 3 times daily.
Topical: Recommended application is for children ages 2-12. To be applied only by a trusted adult or under adult supervision.

Seedlings™ Baby Products

Your baby's health is safeguarded with all-natural, plant-derived formulas in the Seedlings™ product line. Gentle essential oils add a calming effect that enriches your baby's bathing experience.

Seedlings™ Baby Lotion

Keep your baby's skin soft and hydrated with this baby lotion made from plant-based, naturally derived ingredients. You will also love the calming influence of its Lavender-infused essential oil blend.

Ingredients: water, caprylic/capric triglyceride, glycerin, glyceryl stearate, coco-caprylate, cetearyl alcohol, sodium stearoyl glutamate, glyceryl caprylate, xanthan gum, cellulose gum, apple fruit extract, sodium levulinate

Essential Oils: Lavender, Coriander, Bergamot (Furocoumarin-free), Ylang Ylang, Geranium

Directions: Apply a small amount to your hands. Rub hands together to warm the lotion and gently massage into baby's skin.

Caution: *To be applied only by a trusted adult. Keep out of reach of children. For external use only. Discontinue use if skin irritation occurs.*

Seedlings™ Baby Oil

Your baby's delicate skin will thrive with this naturally derived, plant-based formula. With no mineral oil or dangerous phthalates, Seedlings™ Baby Oil nourishes baby's skin while providing the calming scent of appropriately diluted, pure essential oils.

Ingredients: caprylic/capric triglyceride, apricot kernel oil, safflower seed oil, prickly pear seed oil, mixed tocopherols

Essential Oils: Lavender, Coriander, Bergamot (Furocoumarin-free), Ylang Ylang, Geranium

Directions: Apply a small amount to your hands. Rub hands together to warm the oil and gently massage into baby's skin.

Caution: *To be applied only by a trusted adult. Keep out of reach of children. For external use only. Discontinue use if skin irritation occurs.*

Essential Oils Quick Reference Guide

KIDS

Seedlings™ Baby Wash & Shampoo

Gentle and mild, Young Living's Seedlings™ Baby Wash & Shampoo is 100 percent plant based. Your baby's tender skin will be cleansed without overdrying. The calming essential oil blend adds a light and calming scent to enrich baby's bathing experience.

Ingredients: water, sodium laurylglucosides hydroxypropylsulfonate, glycerin, decyl glucoside, glyceryl caprylate, xanthan gum, sodium chloride, sodium levulinate, glyceryl undecylenate, marigold flower extract, caprylic/capric triglyceride, eyebright extract

Essential Oils: Lavender, Coriander, Bergamot (Furocoumarin-free), Ylang Ylang, Geranium

Directions: Wet hair and skin with warm water. Apply a small amount to a moistened washcloth or hand and gently lather over entire body and scalp. Caution: *To be applied only by a trusted adult. Keep out of reach of children. For external use only. Discontinue use if skin irritation occurs.*

Seedlings™ Baby Wipes

These soft, thick wipes do double-duty for diaper changes and feeding clean-ups. Formulated with cleansing botanicals and without harsh chemicals, this baby-safe essential oil blend leaves a delicate, calming scent. Dermatologist tested and hypoallergenic for worry-free care.

Ingredients: water, glycerin, phenethyl alcohol, apple fruit extract, soapberry fruit extract, marigold flower extract, witch hazel leaf extract, caprylic/capric triglyceride, aloe vera leaf juice

Essential Oils: Lavender, Coriander, Bergamot (Furocoumarin-free), Ylang Ylang, Geranium

Directions: Close lid firmly after each use to keep moist. Do not flush. Store at room temperature. Caution: *To be applied only by a trusted adult. For external use only.*

KIDS

Seedlings™ Diaper Cream

With 100 percent naturally derived ingredients, Seedlings™ Diaper Cream provides extra-gentle protection when used at the first sign of diaper rash. It soothes redness, protecting baby's tender skin.

Active Ingredient: non-nano zinc oxide

Ingredients: coconut oil, beeswax, castor oil, mango butter, sunflower oil, safflower oil, cocoa butter, arrowroot, avocado oil, murumuru butter, glyceryl rosinate, kaolin, tocopherol, tamanu oil, grape seed oil, sea buckthorn seed oil, glyceryl oleate, olive oil, and more

Essential Oils: Lavender, Northern Lights Black Spruce, Helichrysum

Directions: Change wet and soiled diapers promptly. Cleanse the diaper area and allow to dry. Apply cream liberally with each diaper change, especially at bedtime or anytime when exposure to wet diapers may be prolonged.

Caution: *For external use only. When using this product, do not get into the eyes. Stop use and ask a doctor if condition worsens, symptoms last more than seven days, or clear up and occur again within a few days.*

Seedlings™ Linen Spray

Capture the clean-air freshness of clothes drying in the sun with this alcohol-free spray, made with 100 percent naturally derived ingredients. Crib sheets, blankets, even car seats can be freshened with the calming aroma of the essential oils in this formula.

Ingredients: water, glyceryl caprylate, glycerin, caprylyl/capryl glucoside, sodium levulinate, glyceryl undecylenate, sodium anisate, sodium cocoyl glutamate, polyglyceryl-5 oleate, caprylic/capric triglyceride, citric acid

Essential Oils: Lavender, Coriander, Bergamot (Furocoumarin-free), Ylang Ylang, Geranium

Directions: Shake well before each use. Spray on linens as needed. Do not spray directly on skin or face.

Caution: *To be applied only by a trusted adult. Keep out of reach of children. For external use only. Discontinue use if skin irritation occurs. Avoid use on fabrics and other materials that may be stained by water.*

HEALTHY & FIT

You work hard to eat a healthy diet and get regular exercise, and we strive to make products that support that effort.

NingXia Nitro™

NingXia Nitro™ is an all-natural way to increase cognitive alertness, enhance mental fitness, promote energy, and support overall performance. Its benefits are derived from a wide range of powerful cognitive enhancers like wolfberry seed oil, combined with therapeutic-grade essential oils. It improves physical performance, speeds up recovery, and increases overall energy reserves, while avoiding the typical caffeine crash.

Ingredients: niacin (as niacinamide), vitamin B6 (as pyridoxine HCl), vitamin B12 (as methylcobalamin), iodine (as potassium iodide), Proprietary Nitro

Essential Oils: Spearmint, Peppermint, Nutmeg, Black Pepper

Directions: Consume directly from the tube or mix with 2-4 oz. NingXia Red®, 1 can of NingXia Zyng™, or 4 oz. water anytime you need a pick-me-up. Best served chilled. Shake well before use.

Allergen Warnings: Contains milk and tree nut (coconut). Not recommended for children.

NingXia Red® (Juice)

Ningxia wolfberries have long been treasured in the natural health community. Their phytochemical profile is legendary: amazing polysaccharides, calcium, 18 amino acids, 21 trace minerals, beta-carotene, vitamins B1, B2, B6, and E, along with polyphenols.

Ingredients: sodium, proprietary NingXia Red® Blend: [whole Ningxia wolfberry puree, blueberry juice from concentrate, plum juice from concentrate, cherry juice from concentrate, and more

Essential Oils: Grape, Orange, Yuzu, Lemon, Tangerine

Directions: Drink 1-2 fl. oz. 1-2 times daily. Best served chilled. Shake well before use. Refrigerate after opening and consume within 30 days.

NingXia Zyng™

NingXia Zyng™ is a light, sparkling beverage that delivers a splash of hydrating energy. It is fueled by a proprietary blend of pure Black Pepper and Lime essential oils, wolfberry puree, and white tea extract, combined with vitamins to create a unique, delicious, and refreshing beverage.

Ingredients: carbonated water, organic cane sugar, pear juice concentrate, wolfberry puree, citric acid, blackberry juice concentrate, natural flavor, white tea leaf extract, stevia rebaudiana leaf extract, and more

Essential Oils: Black Pepper, Lime

Directions: Invert can once before opening.

Ningxia Wolfberry (Organic Dried)

The Ningxia wolfberry is one of earth's most powerful antioxidant fruits. It is rich in polysaccharides, with more vitamin C than oranges, more beta-carotene than carrots, and more calcium than broccoli. These little, red Ningxia wolfberries are delicious and make a great, healthy snack. They can be used in cooking, salads, desserts, etc. The people in Inner Mongolia, where the Lycium barbarum species grows, drink wolfberry tea throughout the day and consume no less than 1-2 oz. daily.

Ingredients: Ningxia Organic Dried Wolfberries

Directions: Keep in a cool, dark place. Chew them, add them to oatmeal and pancakes, mix them in salads, make jams and jellies with them, or mix them with nuts and other dried fruit to make your own trail mix.

Slique® Essence™

Slique® Essence™ combines Grapefruit, Tangerine, Lemon, Spearmint, and Ocotea with stevia extract in a unique blend that supports healthy weight-management goals. These ingredients work together to help control hunger,* especially when use in conjunction with Slique® Tea or the Slique® Complete Kit.

Ingredients: Essential Oils [Grapefruit, Tangerine, Spearmint, Lemon, Ocotea], stevia (rebaudiana)

Directions: Shake vigorously before use. Add 2-4 drops to 4-6 oz. of your favorite beverage, Slique® Tea, or water. Use between and during meals regularly throughout the day whenever hunger feelings occur.

Aromatic: Direct inhalation preferred.

Slique® Tea

Slique® Ocotea Oolong Cacao Spice Tea is a delicious, premium blend of wholesome and rare ingredients. It offers a natural alternative to sugar-laden fruit drinks from concentrates, sodas, and coffees and can be used as part of a healthy weight-management program.

Ingredients: jade oolong tea, inulin, ocotea leaf, Ecuadorian cacao powder, Sacred Frankincense™ powder, natural stevia extract

Essential Oil: Vanilla

Directions: Bring 8 oz. of water to a rolling boil; let cool for 3½ minutes. Place 1 pouch in a cup, mug, or filter and add water. Steep for at least 3 minutes. Use daily before and after workouts, with meals, or anytime you need a natural boost.

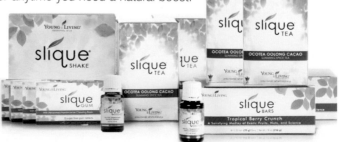

Slique® Shake

Slique® Shake is a complete meal replacement high in protein that helps maintain lean muscle mass and promotes satiety to support your healthy weight-management goals when combined with a sensible diet and regular exercise. This vegan-friendly shake is infused with the Slique® essential oil blend and includes essential dietary fibers and proteins that combine satisfying nutrition with a great berry taste.

Ingredients: pea protein isolate, isomalto-oligosaccharide, medium chain triglycerides, tapioca dextrose, organic coconut palm sugar, natural flavor, organic quinoa powder, organic pumpkin seed protein, and more

Essential Oils: Slique® Essence™ essential oil blend: Grapefruit, Tangerine, Spearmint, Lemon, Ocotea

Directions: Add one Slique® Shake packet to 8 ounces of water or milk of your choice. Shake, stir, or blend until smooth. Fruit, vegetables, or essential oils may be added for additional variety or to enhance flavor.

Slique® Bars—Chocolate-Coated & Tropical Berry Crunch

Safe, innovative, vegetarian weight-management bars that help you feel full sooner and longer, moderate cravings, and provide healthy calories and essential nutrition.

Ingredients: organic Ecuadorian dark chocolate (cane sugar, chocolate liquor, cocoa butter, soy lecithin, vanilla extract), baru nuts, almonds, honey, chicory root inulin, dates, coconut, cacao nibs, goldenberries, Bing cherries, wolfberries, quinoa crisps, chia seeds, potato skin extract, sea salt, sunflower lecithin

Essential Oils: Vanilla, Orange, Cinnamon Bark

Directions: Consume before or between meals with 12 oz. of water to help control hunger. As with any weight-management product, this formula is designed and intended for use with a sensible program of diet and exercise.

HEALTHY & FIT

Gary's True Grit® Einkorn Flour

Einkorn flour contains only unhybridized einkorn grain that has been milled and packaged for use in all flour recipes. The flour is delicious and exceptionally easy to digest.

<u>Ingredients:</u> whole grain einkorn flour

<u>Allergen Warnings:</u> Contains einkorn wheat. Manufactured in a facility that also processes tree nuts, peanuts, soy, milk, and eggs.

Gary's True Grit® Einkorn Granola

Einkorn granola is a tasty combination of crunchy einkorn clusters and a variety of nuts, berries, and seeds packed with energy, a sophisticated flavor, and a symphony of textures. It is made with only the finest, carefully selected, and naturally derived ingredients.

- No added colors, flavors, or preservatives
- No high fructose corn syrup
- Non-GMO ingredients
- Made with whole grains
- Vegan recipe

<u>Ingredients:</u> oats, whole grain einkorn flour, syrup (from fruit juice and grain dextrin), sunflower oil, sunflower seeds, coconut sugar, cranberries, almonds, wolfberries, walnuts, pecans, cacao nibs, vanilla extract, sea salt, Saigon cinnamon

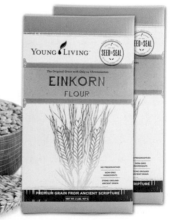

Gary's True Grit® Einkorn Berries

Gary's True Grit® Einkorn Berries bring you all the goodness of the original, non-GMO grain with only 14 chromosomes compared to modern, hybridized wheat, which contains 42 chromosomes.

<u>Ingredients:</u> Contains ancient grain einkorn berries with no preservatives

<u>Directions:</u> Can be ground into traditional einkorn flour or cooked for a hot cereal or spring salad. One cup of einkorn berries will make 1½ cups of ground flour.

<u>Allergen Warnings:</u> Contains einkorn wheat. Manufactured in a facility that also processes tree nuts, peanuts, soy, milk, and eggs.

Supplements
Balance Complete™

Balance Complete™ is a super-food meal replacement that is high in fiber and protein, consisting of good fats, enzymes, vitamins, and minerals needed to form a nutritious, great-tasting protein drink that satisfies the appetite. It is a powerful nutritive energizer and a cleanser, which helps to improve digestion and support colon health.

<u>Ingredients:</u> Proprietary V-Fiber™ Blend: [larch polysaccharides, Ningxia wolfberry fruit powder, brown rice bran, guar gum, konjac, xanthan gum, chicory root fiber extract (FOS), sodium alginate], whey protein concentrate, nonfat dry milk, medium-chain triglycerides, and more

<u>Essential Oil:</u> Orange

<u>Directions:</u> Add 2 scoops of Balance Complete™ to 8 oz. of cold water. May be mixed with rice, almond, or other milk, etc. Shake, stir, or blend until smooth. For added flavor, add fruit or other essential oils.

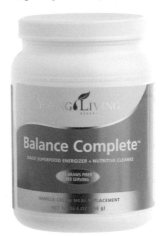

MindWise™

MindWise™ delivers the exotic sacha inchi nut oil and a proprietary blend of pure essential oils and more to support normal brain and cardiovascular function.

Ingredients: vitamin D, proprietary MindWise™

Memory Blend: [pomegranate fruit extract, rhododendron leaf extract, alpha glycerophosphocholine (GPC), acetyl-L-carnitine (ALCAR), coenzyme Q10 (as ubiquinone), turmeric root powder, lithium orotate]

Directions: Drink 1 sachet daily. Consume promptly after opening. Should be taken with a meal. Shake well before each use.

Allergen Warning: Contains tree nuts.

CardioGize™

The perfect combination of heart health and circulation support is found in CardioGize™. Blending vital CoQ10, selenium, and vitamin K2 with supportive herbals results in this superb heart formula.

Ingredients: vitamin K2, folate, selenium, garlic extract, CoQ10, astragalus, dong quai, motherwort, cat's claw, hawthorn berry, cactus powder, cardamom seed powder

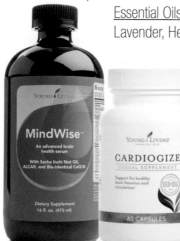

Essential Oils: Angelica, Cardamom, Cypress, Lavender, Helichrysum, Rosemary, Cinnamon Bark

Directions: Take 2 capsules daily. Store in a cool, dark place.

Cautions: Keep out of reach of children. If pregnant or nursing, taking medication, or have a medical condition, consult a health care professional before using.

SAVVY MINERALS
by Young Living™

SAVVY MINERALS
by YOUNG LIVING™

Savvy Minerals by Young Living™ is a cosmetic line formulated exclusively with naturally derived ingredients. It's a pure, toxin-free, mineral-based makeup that is buildable, forgiving, and supportive to the skin. All products are formulated without talc, bismuth, parabens, phthalates, petrochemicals, nanoparticles, synthetic fragrances, synthetic dyes, synthetic colorants, or cheap synthetic fillers.

Savvy Minerals by Young Living™

Savvy Minerals by Young Living™ is a cosmetic line formulated exclusively with naturally derived ingredients. It's a pure, toxin-free, mineral-based makeup that is buildable, forgiving, and supportive to the skin. All products are formulated without talc, bismuth, parabens, phthalates, petrochemicals, nanoparticles, synthetic fragrances, synthetic dyes, synthetic colorants, or cheap synthetic fillers.

Caution: *Keep out of reach of children. For external use only. Storage: Keep in a cool, dark place.*

Savvy Minerals by Young Living™ Misting Spray

Directions: Spray brush 2-3 times. Gently tap off excess moisture before twirling brush in the product lid of your choice. Apply mineral makeup to your face in desired area and reapply as needed.

Ingredients: water, glycerin, aloe vera leaf juice, potassium sorbate, sodium levulinate, sodium anisate, trace mineral complex, citric acid, vanilla fruit extract

Essential Oils: Geranium, Bergamot, Copaiba, Cedarwood, Northern Lights Black Spruce, Orange, Lime, Sage, Ocotea, Rose

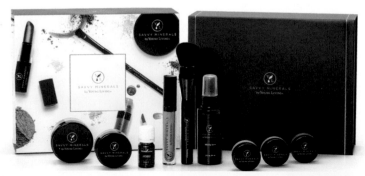

Savvy Minerals by Young Living™ Foundation

The perfect base for a beautiful, natural face. The long-lasting, non-comedogenic formula provides great coverage that actually supports the health of your skin. Using high-quality, mineral-based ingredients, these buildable shades blend flawlessly and provide coverage from light to maximum.

Ingredients: mica, boron nitride, lauroyl lysine, populus tremuloides bark extract, kaolin clay, silica

Directions: Tip the container to sprinkle a small amount of powder into the jar lid. For best results, use a foundation brush. Spray brush 2-3 times with Misting Spray.

Savvy Minerals by Young Living™ Bronzer

Enhance your natural beauty with a healthy, sun-kissed glow any time of year with our mineral bronzer powder. You'll find that Savvy Minerals by Young Living™ Bronzer is great for creating the perfect contour, with a buildable color that blends beautifully.

Ingredients: mica, populus tremuloides bark extract, kaolin clay

Directions: Tip the container to sprinkle a small amount of powder into the jar lid. For best results, use a blush brush. Swirl the brush gently in the lid to pick up the powder. Gently tap off excess over the sink.

Savvy Minerals by Young Living™ Veil

Applies with ease, absorbing excess oil while blurring fine lines and pores for an airbrushed look. Highlight your best features with illuminating Diamond Dust Veil, or set your makeup with a matte finish using our Matte Veil.

Ingredients: mica, populus tremuloides bark extract, kaolin clay

Directions: For best results, apply with a brush. Sprinkle a small amount of Savvy Minerals by Young Living™ Veil onto its jar lid. Dip the brush into the lid to pick up the powder, then lightly tap the brush handle to remove excess.

Savvy Minerals by Young Living™ Blush

Adds a youthful glow that boosts your natural radiance. The finely ground formula provides a smooth, even application that blends perfectly with your natural features. The long-lasting, non-comedogenic formula stays in place to give your cheeks that perfectly natural flush.

Ingredients: mica, populus tremuloides bark extract, kaolin clay

Directions: Tip the container to sprinkle a small amount of powder into the jar lid. For best results, use a blush brush. Swirl the brush gently in the lid to pick up the powder. Gently tap off excess over the sink. Apply to the apples of the cheeks in a circular motion, and blend outward, along the cheekbone toward the temples.

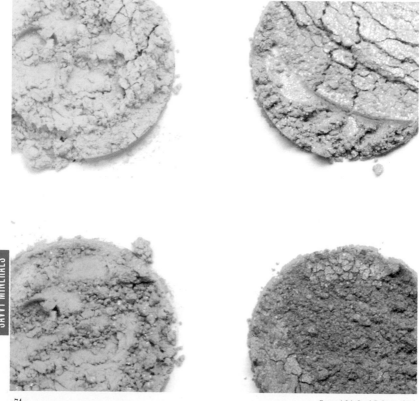

SAVVY MINERALS

Savvy Minerals by Young Living™ Eyeshadow Made with a finely ground mineral base, ensuring they have a smooth, luxurious application. The high-quality-ingredient formula contains no fillers, talc, bismuth, synthetic fragrances, petrochemicals, phthalates, or parabens.

Ingredients: micas, populus tremuloides bark extract, tin oxide

Directions: Tip the container to sprinkle a small amount of powder into the jar lid. For best results, use a blush brush. Swirl the brush gently in the lid to pick up the powder. Gently tap off excess over the sink. Apply to the apples of the cheeks in a circular motion, and blend outward, along the cheekbone toward the temples.

Savvy Minerals by Young Living™ Eyeliner

A natural formula that can be safely applied to the delicate eye area without of toxin exposure to fillers, talc, bismuth, synthetic fragrances, petrochemicals, phthalates, or parabens. It's a great, toxin-free way of creating buildable wet or dry color for looks that range from subtle to the dramatic.

Ingredients: micas, populus tremuloides bark extract, kaolin clay

Directions: For best results, apply with a brush. For everyday wear, wet an eyeliner brush in water and squeeze out any excess, leaving it just damp enough to take up the powder. Dip the brush into the powder, then lightly tap the brush handle against the side of the lid to remove the excess.

Savvy Minerals by Young Living™ MultiTasker A perfect way to enhance your contouring, eyeliner, eyeshadow, brow filler, and even the tone of your foundation. All four colors are made with a finely ground mineral base, ensuring they have a smooth, luxurious application.

Ingredients: micas, populus tremuloides bark extract

Directions: For best results, apply with a brush. Dip the brush into the MultiTasker powder, and then lightly tap the brush handle against the side of the lid to remove the excess. Apply lightly where needed, building and blending color as desired.

SAVVY MINERALS

Savvy Minerals by Young Living™ Poppy Seed Lip Scrub

Formulated to prepare and condition lips so that makeup application is smooth and long-lasting. Savvy Minerals by Young Living™ Poppy Seed Lip Scrub is formulated without parabens, phthalates, petrochemicals, bismuth, talc, synthetic fragrances, or synthetic colorants and is infused with Citrus Fresh™ essential oil blend.

Ingredients: castor seed oil, sucrose, apricot kernel oil, beeswax, cocoa seed butter, shea butter, jojoba esters, papaver somniferum seed, mango seed butter, sweet almond oil, sesame seed oil, silica, avocado butter, glyceryl caprylate

Essential Oils: Orange, Tangerine, Lemon, Grapefruit, Mandarin Orange, Spearmint

Directions: Apply a pea-sized amount to your lips; then exfoliate by massaging in small, circular motions. Use a damp cotton pad to remove. For day, follow with favorite lipstick; for night, follow with a moisturizing lip balm.

Savvy Minerals by Young Living™ Lip Gloss

Provides natural-looking sheer to medium color coverage while adding shine. It's a smooth, flawless application without a sticky finish. Formulated naturally to help moisturize and soften lips, the high level of shine and color can help them look fuller.

Ingredients: castor seed oil, oleic/linoleic/linolenic polyglycerides, beeswax, polyhydroxystearic acid, olive fruit oil, silica, sunflower seed oil, jojoba esters, tocopheryl acetate, tocopherol

Essential Oils: Peppermint

Directions: Apply over the lips alone or with your favorite Savvy Minerals by Young Living™ Lipstick.

SAVVY MINERALS

SAVVY MINERALS by YOUNG LIVING

Foundation

Savvy Minerals by Young Living™ Lipstick

Formulated to bring out every woman's unique and natural beauty. The lipstick glides on smoothly, with a creamy texture and medium coverage that makes application easy and forgiving.

<u>Ingredients:</u> castor seed oil, sweet almond oil, candelilla wax, beeswax, tocopheryl

<u>Directions:</u> Exfoliate lips with Savvy Minerals by Young Living™ Poppy Seed Lip Scrub; then apply a layer of lipstick to deliver nourishing and creamy color. If desired, follow up with a Savvy Minerals by Young Living™ Lip Gloss color of your choice.

Savvy Minerals by Young Living™ Cinnamint-Infused Lipstick

Made to glide on smoothly and add a luxurious shine, this lipstick is full of nourishing ingredients and great natural colors to help you create a bold, impactful look.

<u>Ingredients:</u> castor seed oil, polyglyceryl-2 triisostearate, jojoba seed oil, candelilla wax, coconut oil, lauryl laurate, hydroxystearic/linolenic/linoleic polyglycerides, carnauba wax, shea butter

<u>Essential Oils:</u> Orange, Peppermint, Spearmint, Cinnamon Bark

<u>Directions:</u> Exfoliate lips with Savvy Minerals by Young Living™ Poppy Seed Lip Scrub; then apply a layer of lipstick to deliver nourishing and creamy color. If desired, follow up with a Savvy Minerals by Young Living™ Lip Gloss color of your choice.

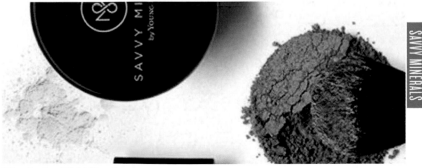

SAVVY MINERALS

Savvy Minerals by Young Living™ Mascara

This natural formula gives lashes a naturally defined look to lashes while conditioning and nourishing them to prevent breakage and encourage growth. The proprietary formula is infused with Young Living's 100% therapeutic-grade Lavender essential oil and includes only naturally derived ingredients.

Ingredients: water, glycerin, hydroxystearic/linolenic/oleic polyglycerides, beeswax, candelilla wax, cetearyl alcohol, pullulan, hydrolyzed jojoba esters, stearic acid, polyglyceryl-10 pentaisostearate, polyglyceryl-6 polyricinoleate, arachidyl alcohol, rice bran wax, glyceryl caprylate, and more

Essential Oils: Lavender

Directions: Comb lashes with the brush in smooth vertical strokes. Apply second coat as needed to reach desired lash volume, length, and separation.

Savvy Minerals by Young Living™ Hydrating Primer

Prep skin for a flawless finish with Savvy Minerals by Young Living™ Hydrating Primer. Help your complexion appear radiant and younger-looking with this hydrating primer. It minimizes the look of pores and fine lines while creating a smooth surface for foundation to adhere to, for long-lasting coverage.

Ingredients: water, coco-caprylate, coconut alkanes, glycerin, brassica campestris/aleurites fordi oil copolymer, shea butter, leuconostoc/radish root ferment filtrate, cocoa seed butter, sodium stearoyl glutamate, and more

Essential Oils: Geranium, Bergamot, Copaiba, Cedarwood, Northern Lights Black Spruce, Orange, Lavender, Lime, Sage, Ocotea, Rose

Directions: Apply a layer of Hydrating Primer to clean, moisturized skin. Allow a few minutes for the primer to set before applying makeup.

Savvy Minerals by Young Living™ Mattifying Primer

Savvy Minerals by Young Living™ Mattifying Primer helps keep shine to a minimum, so the flawless finish of your makeup can last all day. Formulated with Manuka and Tea Tree essential oils, this skin-loving primer gives oily skin a matte finish and long-lasting wear to your foundation while helping reduce the appearance of blemishes. Silky to apply, our new mattifying primer helps blur and smooth fine lines and provides an even surface for foundation to adhere to, helping extend the wear of your makeup.

Ingredients: water, caprylic/capric triglyceride, stearyl alcohol, cetyl alcohol, cetearyl alcohol, glyceryl stearate citrate, glycerin, silica, sodium levulinate, benzyl alcohol, glyceryl caprylate, sodium anisate, shea butter, kaolin, sweet almond oil, sodium hydroxide, sodium carbonate

Essential Oils: Manuka, Frankincense, Rosemary, Tea Tree, Geranium, Lavender

Directions: Apply a layer of Mattifying Primer to clean, moisturized skin. Allow a few minutes for the primer to set before applying makeup..

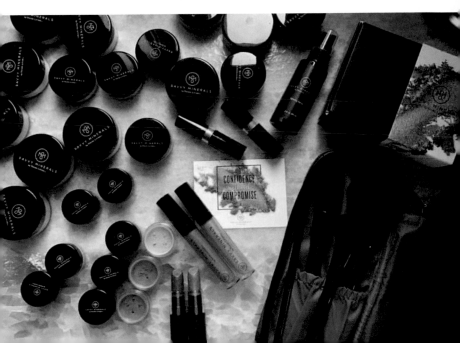

Savvy Minerals by Young Living™ Makeup Remover Wipes

Savvy Minerals by Young Living™ Makeup Remover Wipes are ultra-soft and comfortable. The soothing formula leaves skin moisturized, soft, and smooth while providing gentle and thorough cleansing without drying delicate skin.

Ingredients: water, sorbitan oleate decylglucoside crosspolymer, coco-caprylate, coco glucoside, phenethyl alcohol, coconut alkanes, glyceryl caprylate, isoamyl cocoate, coco-caprylate/caprate, phytic acid, vanilla fruit extract, tocopherol, alcohol, sunflower seed oil, aloe vera leaf juice, althaea officinalis root extract, matricaria flower extract, cucumber fruit extract, oats extract, citric acid

Essential Oils: Geranium, Bergamot, Copaiba, Cedarwood, Northern Lights Black Spruce, Orange, Lavender, Lime, Sage, Ocotea, Rose

Directions: Close lid firmly after each use to keep moist. Do not flush. Store at room temperature.

Savvy Minerals by Young Living™ Solid Brush Cleaner

Savvy Minerals by Young Living™ Solid Brush Cleaner is a gentle formula that cleanses the delicate fibers of Savvy Minerals by Young Living™ brushes. Naturally formulated to provide proper cleaning without harsh toxins—such as chlorine, alcohol, sulfates, parabens, phthalates, mineral oil, animal-derived ingredients, synthetic preservatives, synthetic fragrances, or synthetic dyes.

Ingredients: sodium palmate, sodium palm kernelate, water, glycerin, sodium gluconate, jojoba seed oil, shea butter, moringa oleifera seed oil

Essential Oils: Lavender, Lemon, Orange, Grapefruit

Directions: Wet bar with water before cleansing. Gently rub brush into bar to lather. Place brush under running water with bristles point down until the water runs clear. Reshape brush and lay flat to dry. Allow bar to dry before reusing.

SAVVY MINERALS

AILMENTS

This section lists many common ailments, along with the name of the essential oil and essential oil products that you can use to experience benefits. There is also a brief explanation for the most common and effective application.

This extensive list does not include all possible applications of the essential oils and products. For more information on specific oils or ailments, please see the Essential Oils Desk Reference or visit www.discoverlsp.com. Ailments are listed in alphabetical order; products are listed in recommended order.

ACNE

<u>Products:</u> Melrose™, Purification®, Geranium, Vetiver, Sandalwood, Patchouli, Lavender, German or Roman Chamomile, Melaleuca Quinquenervia, ART® Skin Care System, Mineral Essence™, Detoxzyme
<u>Usage:</u> Apply 3-5 drops neat or diluted 50/50 on affected area 2-4 times daily. Alternate oils, as desired.

ARTHRITIS/JOINT PAIN

<u>Products:</u> PanAway®, Relieve It™, Aroma Siez™, Deep Relief Roll-on, Idaho Balsam Fir, Frankincense, Palo Santo, ICP™, JuvaPower™, Sulfurzyme™, BLM™, Detoxzyme
<u>Usage:</u> Apply 3-5 drops neat or diluted 50/50 on affected area 2-4 times daily. Alternate oils as desired.

ATHLETE'S FOOT/RINGWORM

<u>Products:</u> Melrose™, Thieves®, Purification®, Patchouli, Melaleuca, (M. Alternifolia), Blue Cypress, Lavender, Peppermint, Thyme, Melissa
<u>Usage:</u> Apply 3-5 drops neat or diluted 50/50 on affected area 2-4 times daily. Alternate oils, as desired.

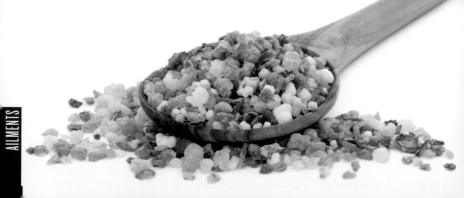

ATTENTION DEFICIT (ADD and ADHD)
Products: Brain Power™, Peace & Calming®, Clarity™, Common Sense™, RutaVaLa™ (oil or roll-on), Vetiver, Lavender, Cedarwood, Peppermint, Frankincense
Usage: Diffuse 15 minutes 4-8 times daily. Massage 3-5 drops on brain stem, back of the neck, and temples.

BACKACHE/LUMBAGO
Products: Aroma Siez™, PanAway®, Relieve It™, Deep Relief Roll-On, Lavender, Idaho Balsam Fir, Wintergreen, Marjoram, Copaiba, Peppermint
Usage: Apply 3-5 drops neat or diluted 50/50 on affected area 2-4 times daily. Alternate oils, as desired.

BLISTERS/BOILS
Products: LavaDerm Cooling Mist, Purification®, Melrose™, Melaleuca (M. Alternifolia), Myrrh, Lavender, Rose Ointment, Spikenard
Usage: Apply 3-5 drops neat or diluted 50/50 on affected every 2-3 hours. Alternate oils, as desired.

BRUISED MUSCLES
Products: German Chamomile, Spikenard, Cistus, Marjoram, Wintergreen, Helichrysum, Cypress, PanAway®, Deep Relief Roll-On, Relieve It™
Usage: Apply 3-5 drops neat or diluted 50/50 on affected area 4-6 times daily.

BUG/INSECT/SPIDER BITES, BEE STINGS, ETC.
Products: Idaho Tansy, Palo Santo, Thieves®, Purification®, Peppermint, Eucalyptus Blue, Dorado Azul, Citronella, Lemongrass, Melrose™, Lavender
Usage: Mix Idaho Tansy and Palo Santo and spray undiluted or mixed with 1/2 cups of water on skin, clothing and bedding. Add 5-10 drops of other oils. Spray Thieves® or Purification® neat or diluted in water. Apply 1-2 drops of chosen oil on area. Your choice of combination.

AILMENTS

BURNS/SUNBURNS

Products: LavaDerm, Cooling Mist, Spikenard, Lavender, Idaho Balsam Fir, Helichrysum, Valor®, Gentle Baby™, Australian Blue™, Melrose™
Usage: Spray as often as needed. Add 3-5 drops of other oil(s) to LavaDerm or other spray mixture as desired and spray or apply 3-5 drops neat or diluted 50/50 on affected area every hour or as needed.

CIRCULATION PROBLEMS (BLOOD)

Products: Helichrysum, Cypress, Tangerine, Idaho Balsam Fir, En-R-Gee™, Aroma Life™, EndoFlex™, Valor® (oil or rub-on), NingXia Red®
Usage: Apply 2-4 drops neat or diluted 50/50 on desired areas. Have a body massage weekly.

COLD SORES (HERPES SIMPLEX TYPE 1)

Products: Melrose™, Purification®, Melissa, Thieves®, Myrrh, Melaleuca (M. Alternifolia), Lavender, Sandalwood, Vetiver, Patchouli, Ravintsara
Usage: Apply 1 drop of chosen oil neat or directly on cold sore every 1-2 hours.

COLDS/FLU/INFLUENZA

Products: Raven™, ImmuPower™, Thieves®, DiGize™, Exodus II™, R.C.™, Mountain Savory, Oregano, Eucalyptus Blue, Peppermint, Clove, Dorado Azul, Inner Defense, Thieves® Mouthwash, Detoxzyme
Usage: Diffuse 30-45 minutes. Inhale directly 2-4 times daily. Apply 3-4 drops neat or diluted on the throat, chest, and back.

CUTS/SCRAPES/WOUNDS

Products: Melrose™, Aroma Life™, Rosemary, Eucalyptus (E. Globulus), Dorado Azul, Thyme, Lavender, Melaleuca (M. Alternifolia), Frankincense, Helichrysum
Usage: Apply 3-5 drops neat or diluted 50/50 on affected area 2-4 times daily. Alternate oils to determine best effect.

AILMENTS

DANDRUFF
<u>Products:</u> Cedar Wood, Rosemary, Melrose™, Thieves®, Citrus Fresh™, Melaleuca (M. Alternifolia), Eucalyptus Blue, Lavender, Lavender Mint Shampoo
<u>Usage:</u> Massage vigorously 1 tsp of desired oil neat or diluted 50/50 into scalp for 2-3 minutes; leave for 15 minutes and then shampoo.

DEPRESSION
<u>Products:</u> RutaVaLa™ (oil or roll on), Hope™, The Gift™, Frankincense, Live with Passion™, Valor® (oil or roll-on), Melissa, Inspiration™, Jasmine, Rose, Mineral Essence, Thyromin, Balance Complete™
<u>Usage:</u> Gently massage 2-3 drops on rim of ears. Diffuse 20-30 minutes 3-4 times daily or as desired. Inhale directly 4-6 times daily.

DIZZINESS/FAINTING
<u>Products:</u> Clarity™, Awaken™, Brain Power™, Common Sense™, Highest Potential™, Grounding™, Ocotea, Eucalyptus Blue, Peppermint, NingXia Red®, MultiGreens
<u>Usage:</u> Apply 1-2 drops neat to the crown, brainstem, and forehead, as needed. Diffuse 30-45 minutes 4-5 times daily. Inhale directly throughout the day, as needed, breathing slowly and deeply.

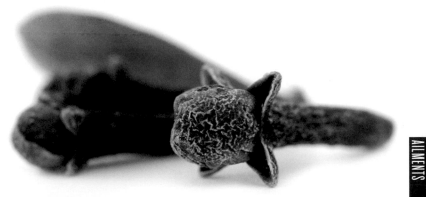

AILMENTS

ECZEMA/DERMATITIS/SKIN DISORDERS

<u>Products:</u> Juva Cleanse®, Purification®, Melrose™, Australian Blue™, Cistus, Blue Cypress, Roman Chamomile, Lavender, German Chamomile, Myrrh, Patchouli

<u>Usage:</u> Apply 4-5 drops neat or diluted 50/50 on affected area, as needed.

EMOTIONAL TRAUMA

<u>Products:</u> Hope™, The Gift™, RutaVaLa™ (oil or roll-on), Trauma Life, Peace & Calming®, Joy™, Inspiration™, Sacred Frankincense™, Valerian, Lavender, Rose, Galbanum

<u>Usage:</u> Diffuse 30-40 minutes 4-5 times daily or as desired. Inhale directly throughout the day, as needed. Apply 1-2 drops neat to the crown, brainstem, and forehead, as needed.

FEVER

<u>Products:</u> Peppermint, Eucalyptus Blue, ImmuPower™, Melrose™, Palo Santo, Spearmint, Orange, Idaho Balsam Fir, Myrrh, M-Grain™, Dorado Azul

<u>Usage:</u> Apply 2-3 drops of neat or diluted 50/50 to forehead, temples, and back of neck.

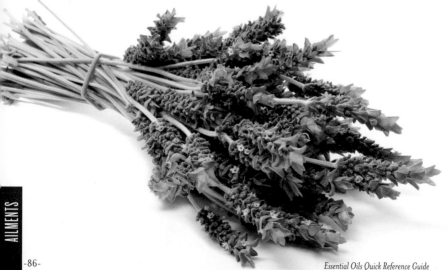

Essential Oils Quick Reference Guide

AILMENTS

FRIGIDITY/SEXUAL DYSFUNCTION

Products: Sclar™Essence, Sensation™, Lady Sclareol™, Mister™, Into the Future™, Motivation™, Valor®, Joy™, Ylang Ylang, Jasmine
Usage: Inhale directly, as desired. Apply 1-2 drops neat or diluted 50/50 on neck, shoulders, and lower abdomen 1-3 times daily.

GUM DISEASE

Products: Thieves®, Melrose™, PanAway®, Thieves® Dentarome Toothpaste, Thieves® Mouthwash, Clove, Peppermint, Melaleuca (M. Alternifolia), Thyme
Usage: Gargle with chosen oil, as needed.

HALITOSIS/BAD BREATH

Products: Thieves®, Purification®, DiGize™, Peppermint, Lemon, Spearmint, Cassia, Ocotea, Essentialzyme, Detoxzyme, Digest & Cleanse, Life 9™
Usage: Gargle 2-4 times daily, as needed. Put 1-2 drops on tongue, as desired.

HEADACHE

Products: M-Grain™, PanAway®, Brain Power™, Clarity™, Deep Relief Roll-On, Stress Away™ Roll-On, Dorado Azul, Eucalyptus Blue, Roman Chamomile, NingXia Red®, ComforTone, Essentialzyme
Usage: Apply 1-3 drops neat or diluted 50/50 on back of neck, behind ears, on temples, on forehead, and under nose. Diffuse 15-30 minutes 3-5 times daily. Inhale directly 3-8 times daily, as needed.

HIGH BLOOD PRESSURE (HYPERTENSION)

Products: Aroma Life™, Peace & Calming®, Ocotea, Lavender, Ylang Ylang, RutaVaLa™ (oil or roll-on) Essentialzyme, OmegaGize3®, CardiaCare, Mineral Essence, Citrus Fresh™
Usage: Dilute body massage daily. Diffuse daily.

* Please refer to Essential Oils Desk Reference for complete usage instructions.

-87-

AILMENTS

HIVES

Products: Myrrh, German Chamomile, Ravintsara, Lavender, RutaVaLa™ (oil or roll-on) Stress Away™ Roll-On, Peace & Calming®

Usage: Apply 2-4 drops neat or diluted 50/50 on location, as needed.

INSOMNIA

Products: RutaVaLa™ (oil or roll-on), Peace & Calming®, SleepEssence, Valor® (oil or roll-on), Stress Away™ Roll-On, Lavender, Cedar Wood, Valerian

Usage: Apply neat 1-3 drops to shoulders, stomach, and on bottoms of feet. Diffuse 30 minutes at bedtime.

LIVER CLEANSING

Products: JuvaFlex™, Ledum, Celery Seed, Lemon, Orange, Rosemary, Juva Cleanse®, Release™, Detoxzyme, JuvaPower, German Chamomile, ComforTone

Usage: Place warm compress over the liver 1 time daily for 15-30 minutes.

MUSCLE CRAMPS/SPASMS

Products: PanAway®, Relieve It™, Aroma Siez™, Rosemary, Marjoram, Vetiver, Deep Relief Roll-On, Ortho Ease and Ortho Sport Massage Oils, MegaCal, Mineral Essence

Usage: Massage 2-4 drops neat or diluted 50/50 on cramped muscle 3 times daily. It may help to alternate cold and hot packs on affected muscle.

NAUSEA/MOTION SICKNESS

Products: DiGize™, Juva Cleanse®, GLF™, Ginger, Nutmeg, Ocotea, Peppermint, AlkaLime, Detoxzyme, Essentialzyme, Spearmint, Valor® (oil or roll-on), Patchouli

Usage: Massage 1-3 drops neat or diluted 50/50 behind each ear and over naval 2-3 times hourly. Put 1 drop on tongue 1-3 times daily or as needed. Inhale directly 4-6 times hourly, as desired.

Essential Oils Quick Reference Guide

AILMENTS

PAIN

Products: PanAway®, Deep Relief Roll-On, Relieve It™, Aroma Siez™, Peppermint, Dorado Azul, Palo Santo, Idaho Balsam Fir, Valerian, Ortho Sport Massage Oil

Usage: Apply 2-4 drops neat or diluted 50/50 on location, as needed.

PARASITES

Products: ParaFree, Thieves®, DiGize™, Juva Cleanse®, Lemongrass, Tarragon, Anise, Basil, ICP, ComforTone, Detoxzyme, Life 6™

Usage: Place a warm compress over intestinal area 2 times weekly.

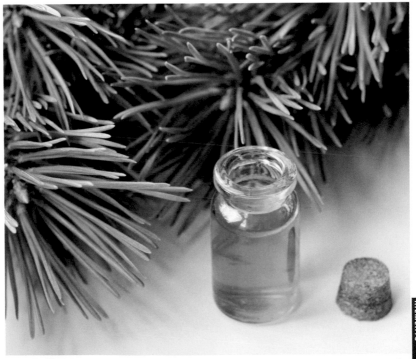

Please refer to Essential Oils Desk Reference for complete usage instructions.

AILMENTS

PMS/MENSTRUAL AND HORMONE CONDITIONS

<u>Products:</u> SclarEssence™, Dragon Time™, EndoFlex™, Lady Sclareol™, Rose, Progessence Plus Serum (1-2 drops on neck or as directed), Prenolone Plus Body Cream, Clary Sage, Fennel, Ylang Ylang

<u>Usage:</u> Apply 4-6 drops neat or diluted 50/50 on the forehead, crown of head, soles of feet, lower abdomen, and lower back 1-3 times daily. Inhale directly throughout the day, as desired.

PNEUMONIA/BRONCHITIS

<u>Products:</u> Raven™, Melrose™, R.C.™, Thieves®, Exodus II™, Thyme, Ravintsara, Eucalyptus (E. Radiata), Oregano, Inner Defense™, Breathe Again™ Roll-On, Super C (or chewable), Mountain Savory

<u>Usage:</u> Diffuse different oils for 15-30 minutes 3-8 times daily. Inhale directly 5-10 times daily, as needed, alternating oils. Apply 2-6 drops neat or diluted 50/50 over neck, back, and chest as needed.

RESTLESS LEG SYNDROME

<u>Products:</u> Aroma Siez™, Peace & Calming®, RutaVaLa™ (oil or roll-on), Stress Away™ Roll-On, Mineral Essence, Basil, Marjoram, Lavender, Cypress, Roman Chamomile, Valerian

<u>Usage:</u> Massage 6-8 drops of oil neat or diluted 50/50 on the leg 3-4 times daily, as needed. Apply 3-4 drops neat to the Vita Flex points on the feet before retiring.

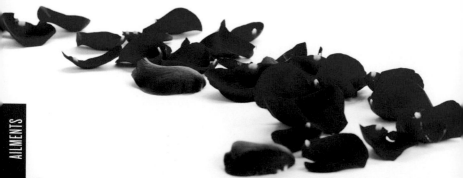

Essential Oils Quick Reference Guide

SHINGLES
Products: Blue Cypress, Australian Blue™, Exodus II™, Thieves®, Elemi, Idaho Tansy, Melaleuca (M. Alternifolia), Lavender, Super Cal, Sulfurzyme, Ravintsara, Melaleuca Quinquenervia
Usage: Apply 6-10 drops neat or diluted 50/50 on affected areas, back of neck, and down the spine 1-3 times daily.

SINUS CONGESTION/INFECTION
Products: DiGize™, Raven™, Thieves®, Exodus II™, Breathe Again™ Roll-On, Peppermint, Eucalyptus Blue, Palo Santo, Eucalyptus (E. Radiata), Ravintsara, R.C.™
Usage: Inhale directly 3-8 times daily, as needed. Put 1-2 drops of oil in water and gargle 3-6 times daily. Massage 1-3 drops neat or diluted 50/50 on forehead, nose, cheeks, lower throat, chest, and upper back.

SORE MUSCLES
Products: PanAway®, Deep Relief Roll-On, Aroma Siez™, Relieve It™, Dorado Azul, Copaiba, Wintergreen, Marjoram, Peppermint, MegaCal, Mineral Essence, Ortho Ease and Ortho Sport Massage Oils
Usage: Massage sore muscles oil neat or diluted 50/50. Apply a warm compress on location.

SORE THROAT/COUGH
Products: Thieves®, Thieves® Lozenges, Thieves® Spray, Eucalyptus (E. Radiata), Lemon, Peppermint, Super C (or chewable), Exodus II™, Ocotea, Eucalyptus Blue, Dorado Azul, R.C.™
Usage: Put 1 drop on the tongue 2-6 times daily. Gargle 4-8 times daily. Inhale directly 3-6 times daily. Apply 1-3 drops neat or diluted 50/50 on throat, chest, and back of neck 2-4 times daily.

SPRAIN/MUSCLE INFLAMMATION

<u>Products:</u> PanAway®, Aroma Siez™, Deep Relief Roll-On, Relieve It™, Wintergreen, Idaho Balsam Fir, Helichrysum, Mineral Essence, Peppermint, Lavender, BLM

<u>Usage:</u> Apply 4-6 drops neat or diluted 50/50 on location 3-5 times daily. Apply a cold compress on location 2 times daily.

STREP THROAT

<u>Products:</u> Exodus II™, Melrose™, Thieves®, Eucalyptus (E. Globulus), Inner Defense, ImmuPro, Frankincense, Super C (or chewable), Myrrh, Dorado Azul, Eucalyptus Blue

<u>Usage:</u> Put 1 drop on the tongue 2-6 times daily, as needed. Gargle 4-8 times daily. Inhale 3-6 times daily. Apply 1-3 drops neat or diluted 50/50 on throat, chest, and back of neck 2-4 times daily.

STRESS/FATIGUE

Products: RutaVaLa™ (oil or blend), Stress Away™ Roll-On, Peace & Calming®, Valor®, Lavender, Valerian, MultiGreens, Power Meal, NingXia Red®, Sandalwood

Usage: Inhale directly as needed. Diffuse 30-45 minutes 1-3 times daily. Apply 2-3 drops on temples, neck, and shoulders 2 times daily or as needed.

URINARY/BLADDER INFECTION

Products: K & B, ImmuPro, Myrrh, EndoFlex™, R.C.™, Melrose™, Thieves®, Spikenard, AlkaLime, Inspiration™, Rosemary, Juniper, Oregano, DiGize™

Usage: Apply a warm compress for 15-20 minutes over bladder area 1-2 times daily.

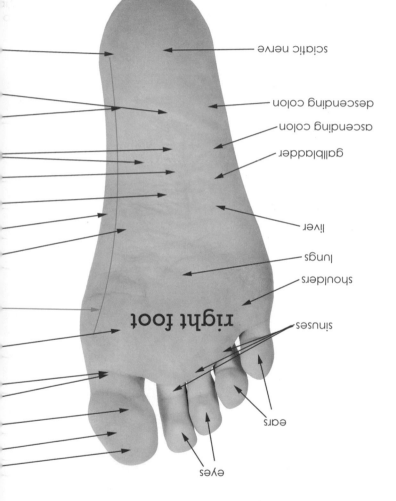

right foot

sciatic nerve

descending colon

ascending colon

gallbladder

liver

lungs

shoulders

sinuses

ears

eyes

* Please refer to Essential Oils Desk Reference for complete usage instructions.

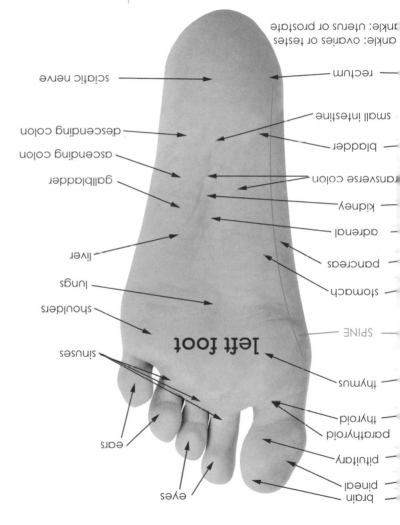

left foot

- rectum
- ankle: ovaries or testes
- ankle: uterus or prostate
- sciatic nerve
- small intestine
- descending colon
- bladder
- ascending colon
- transverse colon
- gallbladder
- kidney
- liver
- adrenal
- pancreas
- lungs
- stomach
- shoulders
- SPINE
- sinuses
- thymus
- ears
- thyroid
- parathyroid
- pituitary
- eyes
- pineal
- brain

Enjoy the benefits of being a…

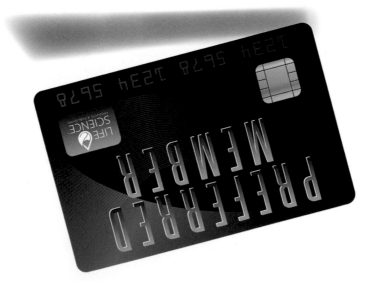

· **80% off** select Shipping!
· Discounts on all products
· Up to **50% off** select items

1.800.336.6308

www.DiscoverLSP.com

LIFE SCIENCE
PRODUCTS & PUBLISHING